Synthetic Children

Synthetic Children

Finding Health in Our Toxic World

DK Guyer, PhD

Scotland Media Group
3583 Scotland Road, Building 70
Scotland, PA 17254

Paperback - 978-1-941746-34-9
eBook - 978-1-941746-35-6

For Worldwide Distribution, Printed in the United States of America

1 2 3 4 5 6 7 / 20 19 18 17

Disclaimer from the Author

These statements have not been evaluated by the Food and Drug Administration. The products mentioned in this book are not intended to diagnose, treat, cure or prevent any disease.

Only a licensed medical doctor can prescribe medical treatment. I am not a medical doctor and do not practice as a doctor; therefore, the content of this book must be disclosed to you as only my opinions, my thoughts, my observations, my conclusions, and serves only as informational and educational material. It is not intended as medical advice, medical diagnosis, or medical treatment.

All people involved in the publishing and distribution of this book are aware that its contents are only for informational and educational purposes. I am not prescribing medical treatment nor am I attempting to negate your current medical treatment plan. Should you choose to follow any of my recommendations, without the supervision of a medical doctor, you are doing so at your own risk.

Natural health protocol is information and education the medical community, pharmaceutical companies, fast food giants, and purveyors of synthetic foods and ingredients do not want you to know.

Should you decide to implement any of the information in this book, you so do at your own risk and are solely responsible for any outcome.

Contents

Acknowledgments

Natural health educators and activists have paved the way for all of us for many years. I am grateful to have learned from some of the most dedicated professionals and enthusiasts from around the globe. I especially wish to thank Dr. Paul Fanny and Dr. Joe Brown for sharing their knowledge and passion for natural health, not only with me, but with the world.

Clients and students, who changed their health for the better after attending one of my classes or seminars, encouraged me to publish a book. To all of you, I offer my sincerest gratitude for believing in me and my message.

The unwavering kindness of my husband, Dale, and my children, Delanie Polca and Jorgan Strathman, helped me remain focused regardless of the obstacles and life's busy schedule. I am blessed with their love every day and so grateful for their encouragement.

To the most wonderful customers in the world: the wholesale and retail clients of Gardens by Grace, LLC. To all of you, I convey my deepest appreciation for your continued patronage and inspiration! Your personal journeys helped forge some of these pages.

A very special thank you to Stephanie Hollada and Daniel Reed for helping change lives one at a time and for offering immeasurable support.

Thank you to Dean Drawbaugh and Scotland Media Group for their superb guidance and expertise.

And, thank you, for embracing this manuscript and exploring the options for better health. Each new day brings an opportunity to share love and laughter and knowledge with yet another person.

Preface

It seems part of our daily routine to hear another story about someone struggling for life battling cancer or a rare form of disease. The pages of social media alert their encompassing world that prayer and positive thoughts and energy are needed for the loved ones fighting for their lives.

The story begging to be told and shared with everyone is how people living in the United States are being transformed from a strong-willed, healthy, brilliant society of people into "synthetic children"—parented by the masterminds of marketing. We are being led to believe that the food purchases we make are safe and aid our health, when the truth reveals that our choices are the opposite—much of our food is unsafe and creates disease.

I believe that illness begins and ends with the marketing strategies of large corporations. From the first sip of soy-based infant formula, containing as much estrogen as five birth control pills, to the first bite of baby food and artificial flavored juices and snacks, you are being groomed for disease.

The process continues with the daily consumption of synthetic and contaminated foods, artificial sweeteners and cholesterol-laden foods until it eventually emerges as a life-threatening disease requiring you to forfeit all the wealth you have spent a lifetime accumulating, to purchase synthetic and chemical medications from the same corporations that helped you acquire the disease.

We have become "synthetic beings" rather than human beings. Nature has provided a bounty of nutritious foods. Yet, our corporate fathers and mothers have altered the value of these foods through genetic modification, insecticides, and a variety of more than 3,000 other chemicals. When we consume these foods, our bodies begin to break down and develop disease. The fact that the United States of America is considered a superpower in the world does not negate the fact that our human bodies are merely that—human. We are a 10,000-year-old model of human beings requiring wholesome nutrition to sustain our lives and protect us from disease.

There is such an astounding sense of negligence and ignorance surrounding real health and nutrition. In a time when corporations profit more from a sick population rather than a healthy population, I feel an overwhelming sense of urgency to inform everyone how simple it can be to become healthy and stay healthy.

As I watch people die of cancer and other debilitating diseases who could have lived through natural health education, it is difficult to bear. These incredible people did not have to die so soon. They were unaware of a different way of life and another option for eradicating disease. Witnessing the devastating grief of those left behind, not knowing there is a way that can limit the progression of disease or eliminate it altogether, creates my urgency to share another option. It is my hope that this information is used and passed along in order to help a loved one or friend.

Death is final; there are no second chances to make better decisions. The world needs to know now that synthetic products are creating gene mutations, feeding deadly diseases, and destroying people's health.

At some point in your lifetime, someone who means the world to you will receive the distressing news of a life-threatening medical condition. Perhaps, it may even be you. Knowing the requirements for maintaining a healthy existence may make a difference when you are contemplating critical decisions about the immediate future for your health or the health of a loved one.

It is my hope that this book will give you the background information you need to make informed choices about your health. Although it is important to seek medical attention when needed, the final decisions made about your health are yours and yours alone. It is not anyone else's right to pressure you into a certain kind of treatment, especially if there are other options. This book reveals what your options are, and how, when faced with tough decisions, you can make those decisions with a level of self-assurance you may not have had previously.

If you have a desire to know more about natural health and want to become more informed and educated, this book is for you. It is full of easy-to-read and understand information and is designed to assist you with making informed choices about maintaining good health.

We have become synthetic children. Sharing the knowledge of natural health, we can help protect a multitude of precious lives.

1

How Your Body Works

Your body is a 10,000-year-old design: the most amazing machine ever to exist! It consists of billions of cells that are deliberately programmed to fight in order to stay alive and operate all the different functions within daily life. The only requirements for this amazing machine—your human body—is pure water, sunlight, fresh air, sleep, relaxation, cleanliness, shelter, exercise, love and emotional support, and nourishment.

In the past five decades, people have begun to view synthetically made foods and medications as acceptable substances to fuel and care for their body. Synthetic foods, however, are not a substitute for natural nutrition. When purchasing a brand-new car, for example, no one would consider putting soda in the gas tank instead of fuel; the vehicle will not operate and it will cause major damage to the engine. If a person were to drink gasoline like a soda, they would not be functioning very well either. Sodas do not belong in cars in the same way gasoline does not belong in people. Everyone knows the requirements for operating their automobile, and hopefully knows not to drink gasoline.

When it comes to fueling the body and maintaining it, people eat anything they want, anytime of the day or night, and expect their bodies to continue functioning properly while disregarding the nutritional requirements for their amazing machine and their good health. We will put synthetic foods in our bodies that are dangerous, like the gasoline, but because it has become a normative part of our society, we do not think twice about the dangerous effects. Cars are replaceable, your body and your health, however, are your most valuable assets.

In this chapter, you will learn how the body digests food and assimilates nutrients, the nutritional requirements for a healthy body, and the important role of water consumption.

Every microscopic speck of your body is made up of living cells preprogrammed to fight for you to stay alive. Each of these cells works in harmony with all the other cells to help you perform countless functions every minute of your life. Providing the cells with the nutrition required to keep them functioning properly creates a foundation for a lifetime of minimal health issues. Learning about nutrition and understanding how the body converts food into nutrients is a fundamental building block of great health.

In early human life, there were no restaurant buffets, people were hunters and gatherers. They ate fresh tree fruits, berries, green vegetables, and herbs early in the day and drank water. Fish and meats were only eaten later in the day after hunting and fishing made them available.

Teas were made from leaves and bark in order to help heal the sick or wounded. Four thousand years ago, herbs and teas were the only medicines available, and eating for optimal digestion was a standard way of life. Herbal remedies were used as the basis for many prescription drugs prescribed today. Human life survived thousands of years through death-defying conditions without all of the university studies and information we have today, because their medicines and food were provided by the Earth.

In today's culture, we are poisoning ourselves by eating all sorts of synthetic foods in disastrous combinations. The body has to work extremely hard to attempt to digest it, revealing a new age of perilous conditions that cause life-long disease and early death. Knowledge is the key to success in anything you attempt to accomplish. Defeating disease and improving your health is a success that is not out of your grasp and can be achieved.

I found the following "history of medicine" that I think is quite profound in a comic yet realistic way:

4,000 Years of Medicine
2000 BC: Here, eat this root.
1000 AD: That root is heathen! Here, say this prayer.
1865 AD: That prayer is superstition! Here, drink this potion.
1935 AD: That potion is snake oil! Here, swallow this pill.
1975 AD: That pill is ineffective! Here, take this antibiotic.
2000 AD: That antibiotic is poison! Here, eat this root.
(Author unknown)

The Digestive Process

Understanding the digestive process is the first step to achieving great health. The digestive system is designed to break down everything we eat and turn it into usable nutriment. The digestive process begins when you chew the food and it is coated with saliva in the mouth. It then travels down the esophagus toward the stomach. Once the food is in the stomach, digestive enzymes begin their function. There are two major digestive enzymes: *pepsin,* a highly acidic digestive enzyme that breaks down the protein into various amino acids; and *hydrochloric acid* that aids in the conversion of carbohydrates into glucose.

Nearly all disastrous health issues result from ignoring the rules of digestion protocol. To most people, eating a cheeseburger or chicken sandwich sounds fairly harmless. That is until you think about how complicated digestion becomes once you put a multi-food group bite into your mouth. Of all the ingredients that go on a cheeseburger, the protein gets digested first. The reason this statement is so important is that protein takes an average of six to twelve hours to digest if food is properly chewed before swallowing. Improperly masticated food results in large pieces of heavy proteins in the stomach, causing longer digestion times.

The average American eats animal protein at nearly every meal, leaving the average American with half-digested proteins in their stomach at any given point in time. Knowing that before the body can give much attention to the remaining stomach contents because it must first attempt to break down the proteins, should cause us to think, *What about the rest of my cheeseburger?* The bread is sitting in your stomach turning into sugar, the lettuce and tomato are rotting, while the cheese is spoiling in your 98.6-degree stomach. Now add in an order of starchy french fries high in carbohydrates and a medium, carbonated water filled with sugar and dyes also known as soda, and all of the sudden the stomach is at maximum capacity, working overtime, and causing discomfort.

Reacting violently under the pressure, the stomach begins secreting more acids to break down all of the food and now, because of lack of space, there is acid nipping at your esophagus, a display we know as acid reflux. This typical fast food lunch syndrome can create not only acid reflux symptoms but heartburn, indigestion, and nausea. Many times, this "stuffed and unsettled" situation is usually counteracted by taking medicine to keep the contents of the stomach settled when the stomach so desperately wants those contents gone.

According to a study by World Resources Institute, "As it stands, the average American diet is the worst in the world, both in terms of overconsumption and waste." Additionally, according to the Organization for Economic Cooperation and Development, "We (Americans) get more of our daily protein intake from animal-based sources than any other country."[1]

We complicate this phenomenon of overconsumption of animal proteins with the fact that the protein being consumed is highly acidic and contaminated! If the only form of nutriment being digested on a daily basis is protein, it is easy to conclude why Americans are overfed, undernourished, and diseased.

Referring to the burger and fries lunch again, because fruits require a different kind of digestive protocol—hydrochloric acid without pepsin—an apple consumed during afternoon break will not be properly digested and assimilated into nutrients. The apple will essentially ferment in the stomach due to the presence of the highly acidic pepsin enzyme still trying to break down the cheeseburger. The apple is now in the stomach with a variety of different proteins waiting to be properly digested.

Understanding that it could take many hours for all the pepsin utilized to digest proteins to become absent from the stomach so that hydrochloric acid can proceed with digesting the carbohydrates from the apple is essential to understanding why people think they are eating a healthy diet. But in fact, they are receiving little to no benefits from their healthy choices due to the sequence they eat the healthy portion of their meals. Once the fermented apple fibers reach the colon, nutrient extraction is inhibited because the correct digestive enzyme was unable to complete its task.

Guidelines for Proper Digestion and Full Nutrient Conversion

The following eating structure is referred to as "Food Combining." In this sequence, the foods you eat can fully digest and properly convert into usable vitamins, minerals, amino acids, and other vital nutrients. When real, whole, non-synthetic foods are consumed, nutrients feed the cells, strengthen muscles and organs, and fortify the immune system, blood, and skin.

Breakfast: Eat fresh, raw fruits. For example, enjoy a variety of berries for several days, then citrus fruits for the remainder of the week. The idea is to eat a wide variety. Purchase the fresh organic fruits on sale that week. There is no need to over-purchase. Buy what you can consume: 3 apples, 3 pears, 2 bananas, 3 oranges, and some grapes. Varying your fruit consumption provides an array of vitamins and minerals and provides enjoyment so you are not bored with your breakfast.

Morning snack: Eat another piece of fresh fruit.

Lunch: Have a large, fresh salad with all the vegetables you like: lettuce, spinach, cucumber, peppers, onions, kale, mushrooms, radishes, carrots, broccoli, cauliflower, beets, and fresh herbs such as parsley, oregano, basil, and rosemary. Vary the combinations to receive the multitude of vitamins and minerals in fresh, raw vegetables. A small serving of a starch is acceptable with the salad. Some choices could be organic whole grain pasta, an oven-baked organic potato or yam, organic hummus, or organic plantain chips.

Afternoon snack, if needed: Fresh vegetables such as carrots or celery.

Dinner: Select lean, fresh organic meat, wild-caught fresh fish, organic eggs, or organic nuts. Enjoy this meal with raw or lightly steamed vegetables. If you are still hungry, eat more of the same protein and any other non-starchy vegetables. Do not mix protein categories (flesh, seafood, nuts or dairy) for optimal digestion.

When you provide your body with sufficient nutrients, you become less likely to get sick.

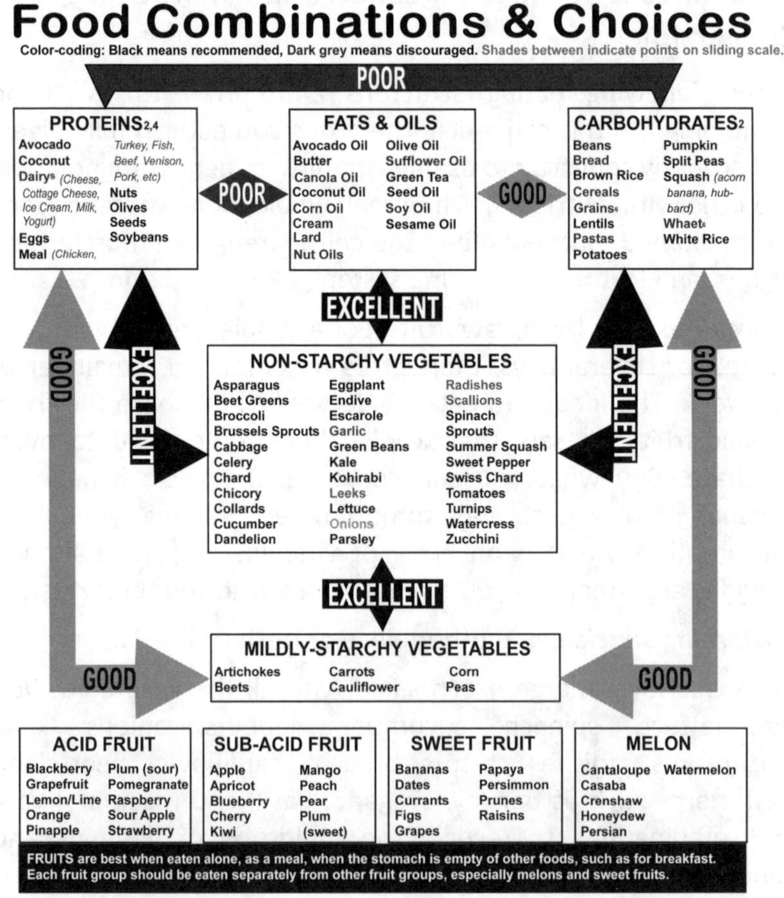

2

Your Body's Nutritional Requirements Protein

The list of nutritional requirements to properly operate your body at an ultimate level is vast. Consuming fresh, raw, organic fruits and vegetables, seeds and nuts supplies the majority of these necessities. Every organ has its own nutritional requirements and each cell demands antioxidants to avoid damage from toxins and other free radicals your body is exposed to in daily life.

In this chapter, you will learn the components of each nutritional category and the role they play in helping your body function properly.

Protein

Proteins are amino acids linked together in long chains. Each specific chain of amino acids helps perform different functions in the body. Some of the functions follow:

- Protein creates antibodies to defend and protect against bacteria and germs.
- Enzymes are created to perform chemical reactions within the cells.
- Proteins are responsible for tissue growth and repair.
- Proteins facilitate communication between cells and organs and your body's actual movements.

Content	Beef	Chicken	Turkey	Eggs*
	Lean	Breast	Leg	
Protein	**49.2**	**29.8**	**27.87**	**13.53**
Calories	**505**	**197**	**208**	**204**
Size	**6 oz**	**100g**	**9.82**	**2 eggs**
Minerals				
Potassium - mg	**393**	**245**	**288**	**168**
Phosphorus - mg	**296**	**214**	**210**	**207**
Calcium - mg	**27**	**14**	**21**	**87**
Magnesium - mg	**32**	**27**	**27**	**15**
Iron - mg	**4.11**	**1.07**	**1.4**	**1.46**
Sodium - mgbe	**80**	**71**	**63**	**342**
Zinc - mg	**11.32**	**1.02**	**2.03**	**1.22**
Manganese - mg	**0.017**	**0.018**	**0.02**	**0.027**
Copper - mg	**0.168**	**0.05**	**0.047**	**0.017**
Selenium - mcg	**45.9**	**24.7**	**29.1**	**27.4**
Also contains a small amount of other minerals.				
Vitamins:				
C - mg				**0.2**
B1-thiamine - mg	**0.1**	**0.066**	**0.057**	**0.063**
B2-riboflavin - mg	**0.291**	**0.119**	**0.131**	**0.533**
B3-Niacin - mg	**6.979**	**12.71**	**6.356**	**0.096**
Pantothenic Acid - mg	**0.971**	**0.936**	**0.634**	**1.229**
B6-Pyridoxine HCl-mg	**0.0481**	**0.56**	**0.48**	**0.144**
Folate - 15 mcg	**15**	**4**	**6**	**37**
B12 - mcg	**3.62**	**0.32**	**0.36**	**0.94**
A - IU	**3.62**	**93**		**642**
E - mg	**0.87**	**0.27**		**1.33**
K - mcg	**3.1**	**0.3**		**4.9**
D - IU	**14**	**5**		**59**
Contains some other vitamins in small amounts.				
*No Salt Added				
Information compiled from Dr. Decuypere Nutrient Charts health-alternatives.com				

Content	Salmon	Almonds	Cashews	Walnuts
	Wild	Raw	Raw	Raw
Protein	**25.44**	**6.02**	**5.17**	**4.32**
Calories	**182**	**163**	**157**	**185**
Size	**100g**	**1 oz**	**1 oz**	**1 oz**
Minerals				
Potassium - mg	**628**	**200**	**187**	**125**
Phosphorus - mg	**256**	**137**	**168**	**98**
Calcium - mg	**15**	**75**	**10**	**28**
Magnesium - mg	**37**	**76**	**83**	**45**
Iron - mg	**1.03**	**1.05**	**1.89**	**0.82**
Sodium - mgbe	**56**		**3**	**1**
Zinc - mg	**0.82**	**0.87**	**1.64**	**0.88**
Manganese - mg	**0.021**	**0.648**	**0.469**	**0.88**
Copper - mg	**0.321**	**0.282**	**0.622**	**0.45**
Selenium - mcg	**46.8**	**0.7**	**5.6**	**1.4**
Also contains a small amount of other minerals.				
Vitamins:				
C - mg			**0.1**	**0.4**
B1-thiamine - mg	**0.275**	**0.06**	**0.12**	**0.097**
B2-riboflavin - mg	**0.487**	**0.287**	**0.016**	**0.043**
B3-Niacin - mg	**10.077**	**0.96**	**0.301**	**0.319**
Pantothenic Acid - mg	**1.92**	**0.133**	**0.245**	**0.162**
B6-Pyridoxine HCI - mg	**0.944**	**0.041**	**0.118**	**0.152**
Folate - 15 mcg	**29**	**14**	**7**	**28**
B12 - mcg	**3.05**			
A - IU	**44**			**6**
E - mg		**7.43**	**0.26**	**0.2**
K - mcg			**9.7**	**0.8**
D - IU				
Contains some other vitamins in small amounts.				
*No Salt Added				
Information compiled from Dr. Decuypere Nutrient Charts health-alternatives.com				

Protein is essential for a healthy body and understanding the different classifications of protein, how much protein to consume, and the benefits or detriments of your choices help you make educated food choices.

Organic red meat contains protein and is typically high in fat, calories, and cholesterol. It takes approximately ten to twelve hours to digest when fully masticated. It does supply vitamin B12, iron, potassium, and other valuable nutrients. Trim the excess fat away before preparing to limit your fat intake and chew it fully before swallowing to assist proper digestion. Due to the high fat and cholesterol constituents of red meat and its associated acidity level, I recommend consuming it in limited quantities: no more than once per week.

Organic poultry, defined as chicken, duck, turkey, and goose, contains protein and supplies vitamins B6 and B12, niacin, and magnesium. While it is lower in calories, fat, and cholesterol than red meat, organic poultry is still acidic in the body. It takes approximately eight to ten hours to digest when fully masticated. Organic poultry is often viewed as a more easily digested animal protein compared to red meat.

Wild-caught fish contains protein but each species offers different nutrients. Albacore tuna, Alaskan salmon, and sardines offer the highest amounts of Omega-3. A diet rich in natural Omega-3 and Omega-6 provides support for a healthy heart. The fish category is not treated equally across all species when it comes to consumption. Only eat wild-caught fish because farm-raised fish are fed an unnatural diet of grains, synthetic foods and chemicals to enhance their color. A portion of these contaminants remain in the fish that you consume.

Avoid shark, mackerel, bluefin tuna, chilean sea bass, grouper and orange roughy due to high mercury content that can cause arthritic conditions. Some safer options when choosing fish include cod, halibut, haddock, flounder, rainbow trout, and tilapia. Most wild-caught fish contain potassium, phosphorus, magnesium, and niacin. Fish is lower in fat, calories, and cholesterol than red meat and poultry. It is an acidic food according to the PRAL list.

Wild-caught seafood is different from its fellow-finned water friends. Seafood is defined as an ingestible water creature having no fins and inhabiting a shell or shell-like structure, commonly known as a crustacean. It includes crab, shrimp, lobster, oysters, clams, mussels, and langostinos. These delicacies are low in calories and fat but are high in cholesterol. Crab contains high enough levels of LDL cholesterol (the bad kind) to consider it as dangerous as red meat. Lobster and shrimp are high in LDL cholesterol as well and should be consumed sparingly. Seafood is not listed on the PRAL (Potential Renal Acid Load) list, but is considered an acidic food.

Organic dry beans should be consumed on a limited basis and only at the evening meal. They contain both protein and carbohydrates making their digestion time of fourteen to sixteen hours excessive by complicating the digestion of other foods present in the digestive process at the same time. Plant-based proteins tend to digest much faster than animal proteins. Beans, depending upon the type and quantity, can impede proper digestion. Beans offer many nutrients and their nutritional categories are vast. Beans are low in fat, calories, and are considered a good source of HDL cholesterol. Green beans are listed as an alkaline food; all other beans are acidic foods.

Eggs can be used as an ingredient in a variety of recipes or prepared as a meal of just eggs. Organic and free-range eggs provide better nutrition than commercially produced conventional eggs. One large free-range egg contains less cholesterol and saturated fat, more vitamins A and E, beta carotene and Omega-3 fatty acids than a conventional egg.[1] Free-range birds consume a more natural diet and benefit from fresh air and sunshine. Organic eggs produce some of the similar increased vitamin components. One commercial egg has more cholesterol than a lean eight-ounce steak. While naturally occurring cholesterol in protein foods does perform a necessary function in the body, managing cholesterol intake to 150 mg-200 mg daily for an active adult will help keep your cholesterol levels in balance. Relatively low in calories and fat, eggs contain a high level of LDL cholesterol when consuming the egg yolk. Eggs are an acidic food—the yolk is twenty-one times more acidic than the egg white. To enjoy the nutritional benefits of eggs, discard some of the yolk and eat the egg whites.

Organic nuts are a good source of protein and natural fats. This category is as diverse as fish; each nut variety offers a different spectrum of valuable nutrients. Almonds are a great source of potassium, magnesium, and vitamin E. Walnuts contain Omega-3, potassium, and the B-complex vitamins. Cashews are an excellent source of selenium. Almonds, Brazil nuts, cashews, hazelnuts, and walnuts can help lower your LDL cholesterol levels. These nuts have zero cholesterol and contain a wide variety of vitamins, minerals, and healthy fats.

Nuts are higher in fats and calories than most people are aware. Even though the fats in nuts are considered healthy, consuming large quantities can aid in weight gain. They are easy to consume, especially when there is little time for food preparation. Organic raw nuts contain more nutrients than roasted or other commercially produced and altered nuts. Nuts are considered an acidic food and should be consumed based on a serving size daily for optimum benefits.

All plant foods contain protein. Each fruit and vegetable offers different vitamin and mineral components. Fruits and vegetables are rarely thought of as a great source of protein. Consuming fresh fruits and vegetables provides ultimate nutrition, low in fat, cholesterol, and calories; these alkaline foods are tasty options for protein consumption that digests in two hours or less.

The following list from the USDA Nutrient Database for Standard Reference, Release 18 shows the protein content expressed in percentage of calories for fruits and vegetables:

Spinach	30%
Asparagus	27%
Lettuce, Green leaf	22%
Broccoli	20%
Kale	16%
Cabbage	15%
Tomatoes, Red	12%
Cucumbers	11%
Apricots	10%
Corn	10%
Peaches	8%
Oranges, Valencia	7%
Strawberries	7%
Watermelon	7%
Carrots	6%
Cherries	6%
Bananas	4%
Grapes, Red	4%

Protein is a building block for the body's daily function. Too much of a good thing, however, is not necessarily the best choice. A high-protein diet, especially high animal protein, is very dangerous!

The low-carbohydrate, high-protein diet craze may have resulted in some weight loss, but it corrupts the body's ability to process much-needed nutrients. In an article written by the Physicians Committee for Responsible Medicine, entitled, "The Protein Myth," excessive protein was considered a detriment to health. The following quote exposes the health complications associated with a high-protein diet: "Excess protein has been linked with osteoporosis, kidney disease, calcium stones in the urinary tract, and some cancers."[2]

Herbs and spices offer protein as well as many other nutritional benefits. They are a tasty alkaline nutrient source with zero cholesterol, zero fat, and are very low in calories.

http://www.pcrm.org/health/diets/vskvegetarian-starter-kit - protein

Herb/Spice	Measure	Protein (g)
Allspice, Ground	1 tsp	.12 g
Anise Seed	1 tsp	.37g
Basil, Dried	1 tsp	.16g
Basil, Fresh	5 leaves	.08g
Caraway Seed	1 tsp	.42g
Cardamom, Ground	1 tsp	.22g
Celery Seed	1 tsp	.36g
Chervil, Dried	1 tsp	.14g
Chili Powder	1 tsp	.36g
Cinnamon, Ground	1 tsp	.10g
Cloves, Ground	1 tsp	.13g
Coriander Leaf, Dried	1 tsp	.13g
Coriander Seed	1 tsp	.22g
Cumin Seed	1 tsp	.37g
Curry Powder	1 tsp	.29g
Dill Seed	1 tsp	.34g
Dill Weed, Fresh	5 sprigs	.03g
Fennel Seed	1 tsp	.32g
Fenugreek Seed	1 tsp	.85g
Garlic Powder	1 tsp	.51g
Ginger, Ground	1 tsp	.16g
Mustard Seed, Ground	1 tsp	.52g
Nutmeg, Ground	1 tsp	.13g
Onion Powder	1 tsp	.25g
Oregano, Dried	1 tsp	.09g
Paprika	1 tsp	.33g
Parsley, Dried	1 tsp	.13g
Pepper, Black	1 tsp	.24g
Pepper, Cayenne	1 tsp	.22g
Pepper, White	1 tsp	.25g
Poppy Seed	1 tsp	.50g
Rosemary, Dried	1 tsp	.06g
Rosemary, Fresh	1 tsp	.02g
Safron	1 tsp	.08g
Sage, Ground	1 tsp	.07g
Savory, Ground	1 tsp	.14g
Spearmint, Dried	1 tsp	.10g
Thyme, Dried	1 tsp	.09g
Turmeric, Ground	1 tsp	.29g
*The USDA Nutrient Database for Standard Reference, Release 28		

High-protein diets can also lead to a variety of health complications including high cholesterol, cardiovascular disease, heart palpitations, and calcium depletion. The recommended protein intake is 10-12 percent of your daily caloric intake. The majority of that protein can be ingested through a variety of organic fresh fruits and vegetables, organic grains, lentils, nuts, seeds, and wild-caught fish.

A high-protein diet does not provide energy. Protein does indeed help build muscle. Excessive protein consumption, however, does not help you build more muscle or build muscle faster. Your body has to process and eliminate the extra protein it does not need and cannot assimilate, placing an incredible strain on the liver, kidneys, and heart.

Protein does not provide energy either. Its primary function is to help grow and rebuild cellular tissue. The higher the protein diet, the higher the risk factor is for disease. Carbohydrates are used for energy and, as stated before, cannot be effectively assimilated into nutrients when consumed with proteins. The more protein you consume, the more fatigue you will experience.

One of the most popular high-protein diets is "The Atkin's Diet." Almost everyone, including medical doctors, natural practitioners, nutritionists, and trainers will agree that when you alter your diet to include more protein and less carbohydrates, you will lose weight. On this diet, lean protein is eaten with vegetables and without carbohydrates. This is the first rule of food combining. The body can properly digest this type of meal, convert the protein and vegetables into nutrition and, because there are no carbohydrates, there are no fats left to store.

The problem with consuming this type of diet beyond three weeks is the lack of nutrients and the amount of protein that the body has to process. The human body requires a variety of nutrition.

Eating three eggs and five pieces of bacon is not healthy. This meal is a heart attack on a plate kind of meal! It is high in protein but outlandishly high in LDL cholesterol. Bacon is listed as a carcinogenic agent with *sufficient evidence* in humans by the World Health Organization.[3] The entirety of this meal is contaminated and extremely difficult to digest. No amount of good health can come from this type of meal.

Let's move on to lunch: A grilled chicken salad with eggs and cheese. This lunch sounds wonderfully healthy to many people, but it is far from making the healthy list. There are three different proteins combined in the same meal that are processed, contaminated, acidic, and high in LDL cholesterol. This meal is not properly food combined, and the few vegetables being consumed from this salad will not negate the negative health effects of the protein consumption. To add to this situation, all the acidic protein from breakfast has not yet been digested.

Dinner time arrives and a steak and broccoli is consumed: another healthy-sounding meal. But the protein from lunch has not yet been digested, breakfast has perhaps just been fully digested, and now more protein is on the way through the digestive system.

Generally, a high-protein diet is acidic, genetically-modified, cooked, dead, dry, fiber-poor, toxic, high in LDL cholesterol, limited in nutrition, highly carcinogenic, very expensive and difficult for the body to digest and process, and just not worth the damage to your health.

It is difficult to find a study that supports a high-protein diet as a lifestyle because it creates disease. Many people are on a high-protein diet because they think it is the best for them. Some instructors at local fitness centers promote the high-protein diet because they think the same thing—not because they possess the education and knowledge of nutrition and how the human body works.

The following information, taken from the "High-Protein Diet Dangers" article by Dr. Russell Blaylock, may help you gain a more complete understanding of the hazards associated with a high protein diet.

> High-protein diets alter special cell-signaling mechanisms that damage cells and shorten lifespan. We are now seeing that this mechanism is playing a major role in many diseases, especially degenerative diseases of the brain. Protein drinks, even those not made from whey, are high in glutamate, which is a major excitotoxin. It also is a powerful promoter of cancer growth and cancer spread.[4]

Discovering the real purpose of protein for bodily functions and good, clean, nutritional sources of protein can help you establish a more balanced diet that will help you reach your weight loss or weight lifting goals without compromising your health. Because advocates of a high protein diet still insist that it is the ultimate food regimen, I need to provide you as much documented proof regarding the very real dangers that exist for loyal followers of high-protein diets.

The following excerpt from the article "Dangers of a High-Protein Diet" by Dr. Agatha Thrash illicits fear when you realize one of the devastating effects of a high-protein diet can take your life.

> Many people are aware of the sudden deaths that occurred because of the unbalanced diet used in weight reduction—a liquid, high-protein, low-carbohydrate diet. The deaths were the result of an irregular rhythm of the heart, caused by such severe derangement in the nutritional balance of the body that proper electrical impulses could not be maintained by the heart.
>
> While sudden death is a dramatic and urgent matter, there are also disabling disorders of a chronic nature that come from a high protein diet. It can be readily stated that a high protein diet is toxic to the body. A high protein diet puts a tax on the liver, breaks down protein tissues, triggers a loss of calcium from bones, and leaves toxic residues which must be eliminated. Before elimination of these toxic residues, however, the body is often damaged so that it is more susceptible to a variety of diseases, including cancer and arthritis.[5]
>
> http://www.ucheepines.org/dangers-of-a-high-protein-diet/

Death is the ultimate price to pay for adopting an unhealthy, high-protein diet. While you may lose a few pounds upon starting a high-protein regimen, the loss of vital nutrients associated with this type of diet establishes windows of opportunity inside your body for disease to gain a stronghold; and with a continued high-protein food focus, that disease can erupt into cancer, stroke, severe heart disease, Alzheimer's disease, and even death.

High-protein diets are prevalent among fitness seekers. I used to work out at the gym about the same time every day or every other day. While there, I witnessed a man stop in the middle of his workout to ingest beef jerky and ostrich sticks. He was preparing for a boxing match, and he announced to everyone in the immediate vicinity that he had to eat protein to maintain his muscle strength. He lost his boxing match because he ran out of energy during the fourth period.

His coach showed up at the fitness center the next week wanting to see his workout because he was so sluggish during the match. The coach's advice to this hardworking, trusting young man was to increase his protein, drink more milk, and start jumping rope. I did not have a degree in natural health at the time, but knew enough about the body to realize the coach's advice was not at all helpful.

The young man collapsed at the fitness center several days after the coach's visit. He was hospitalized, I don't know for how long, and withdrew from boxing. I did not see this man again for several months. When he returned to the fitness center, he was drinking water while working out and I never saw him eating beef jerky or ostrich sticks at the gym again.

Protein is essential for good health. Choose a healthy source of protein. Processed protein powders and protein bars are toxic, synthetic, costly, completely unnecessary, and offer nothing to benefit your better health. If you feel you must have animal protein, please consider consuming only organic meats to eliminate your exposure to contaminated meat products. Eat them only at the evening meal for proper digestion and consume only 10-12 percent of your daily calories in animal protein. Animal protein is difficult to fully masticate, hard to digest, costly, high in LDL cholesterol, acidic, and overall, just not that incredibly healthy for you to be consuming on a daily basis.

When embracing a vegetarian or vegan diet, you should consider enhancing your diet with a quality B12 or B complex supplement to secure the needed B12 that is naturally occurring in meats, eggs, fish, and seafood.

3

Carbohydrates

Carbohydrates are the main source for the body's energy. Fruits and vegetables supply the highest amount of nutrients than any other category of food. The reason you should eat them fresh and raw is because they lose some of their nutritional content during the cooking process. Steaming decreases nutritional value by 15-25 percent, boiling decreases it by 30-40 percent and baking decreases the nutritional value by 30-60 percent, depending on the temperature and length of time in the oven. Bake fruits and vegetables at a temperature of 350 degrees or less to help eliminate total destruction of nutrients.

Natural carbohydrates should account for approximately 80 percent of your daily caloric intake. The majority of carbohydrates should come from fresh fruits and vegetables. Grains should be limited to 10 percent or less of daily calories. Carbohydrates help you create fuel for energy. Fruits and vegetables digest faster and easier than grains, allowing you to quickly fuel and refuel your body.

Many athletes, not just vegetarian and vegan athletes, make it a habit to consume natural forms of carbohydrates before an event for better performance. Protein does not convert into energy in the body but carbohydrates do. Furthermore, carbohydrates in fruit help stimulate the brain, aiding in a clearer mind regardless of your profession. Even if you are not an athlete, you will benefit from fresh fruit and vegetable consumption for your carbohydrate consumption.

Carbohydrates encompass a large selection of foods. Not all carbohydrates offer equivalent nutrition or energy. This is where most of the confusion exists about carbohydrate consumption.

The general mindset is that carbohydrates are bread, rice, pasta, potatoes, and any type of breadstuff. Fruits are carbohydrates, also. The only fruit many people associate with carbohydrates is a banana.

The University of Michigan Comprehensive Diabetes Center designed an easy-to-read and inclusive carbohydrate food chart. This chart lists foods in ten separate categories making it one of my favorite charts to use for educational purposes. Simply by looking at the categories, the reader can quickly learn that carbohydrates are included in many foods and food products. The categories include:

Bread Products	Fruit/Vegetable Juice
Cereal/Bread/Grains/Pasta	Baked Goods
Fruit	Combination Foods
Milk & Yogurt	Sauce & Condiments
Starchy Vegetables	Snack Foods

The full chart can be viewed at www.med.umich.edu1/libr/MEND/CarbList.pdf.

Consuming fresh fruit provides fast and easy digestion that leads to faster conversion to energy inside the body. Other carbohydrates, such as potatoes, pasta and rice, bread, and bakery items, for example, require more time to digest and provide less nutrition. This means that the body will expend more energy digesting these types of carbohydrates, and in return, produce less energy than a fruit or vegetable. You end up spending more energy digesting something that provides less energy and nutrients.

Bananas are the top carbohydrate to consume for optimal energy. They are easy to digest, provide an abundance of minerals, help control blood sugar levels, contain antioxidants and help restore lost electrolytes. Grains, another carbohydrate, cannot accomplish all of that! Neither can protein! Fruits are the ultimate, nutrient-filled carbohydrate.

The following charts are just a sample of some foods containing carbohydrates and understanding the amount of sugar those carbohydrates convert into during digestion, which is sometimes misunderstood. The last column shows the amount of sugar in teaspoons for each carbohydrate on the list.

Fruit	**Size**	**Carbs(g)**	**Tsp Sugar**
Apple	8 oz	30	7.5
Applesauce, unsweetened	1/2 cup	15	3.75
Apricots, dried	7 pieces	15	3.75
Banana	7"	35	8.75
Blackberries/blueberries	1 cup	20	5
Fruit Combo, canned in own juice	1/2 cup	15	3.75
Cantaloupe, Honeydew	1 cup	15	3.75
Cherries	12	15	3.75
Dates, Medjool, dried	1	15	3.75
Grapefruit	1/2 large	15	3.75
Grapes	15	15	3.75
Kiwi	1	15	3.75
Oranges	1	15	3.75
Peaches, canned in own juice	1/2 cup	15	3.75
Pears	6 oz	20	5
Pineapple	1 cup diced	20	5
Prunes	3	15	3.75
Raisins	35	15	3.75
Raspberries	1 cup	15	3.75
Strawberries	1 cup halves	12	3
Watermelon	1 cup diced	12	3

*Adapted from the University of Michigan Comprehensive Diabetes Center Carb List

When fruits are consumed after a work-out, whether it is physical labor on the job or an athletic performance, the energy expended throughout the day is restored faster, which leaves the impact on your muscles less abrasive and apparent.

Fresh, raw, organic fruits and vegetables provide low fat, wholly nutritious, easy-to-digest, high-energy, low-glycemic, low-cholesterol choices for carbohydrate consumption.

Bread, bakery items, cereals, and other processed carbohydrates convert into glucose just like fruits and vegetables. Because of the synthetic components in most of these carbohydrates, they do not provide the same amount of energy.

A donut is considered a carbohydrate by many dieticians. It is not just a carbohydrate. It contains refined sugars, cholesterol, saturated fats, little nutritional value, and a variety of synthetic components. Compare that to an organic apple that is also considered a carbohydrate. It contains natural sugars, zero cholesterol, no saturated fats, no synthetic components, only wholesome nutrition. For this reason, carbohydrates are not all created equally and should not be classified as the same unit of energy when counting carbs for diet or health considerations.

Baked Goods/Snack Foods	**Size**	**Carbs (g)**	**Tsp Sugar**
Cupcake w/frosting	1	30	7.5
Danish-large bakery type	1	45	11.25
Dark Chocolate	1 oz	15	3.75
Donut, plain	1	25	6.25
French Fries-frozen crinkle	10	15	3.75
Ice Cream- vanilla	1/2 cup	15	3.75
Muffins-bakery type	1	65	16.25
Potato chips	1 oz	15	3.75
Pretzels	11 small	15	3.75
Tortilla chips	1 oz	20	5

*Adapted from the University of Michigan Comprehensive Diabetes Center Carb List

When enjoying a delicious muffin from a bakery, you essentially are eating just under three days' worth of sugar content using the rule of 6 teaspoons of sugar per day. The muffin contains harmful ingredients and saturated fat. The 65 grams of carbohydrates for one muffin equates to:

1 cup of strawberries (halved)	12 g carbs
1 cup of raspberries	15 g carbs
1 cup of blueberries	15 g carbs
1 orange	15 g carbs
½ cup of watermelon (diced)	8 g carbs

All of this fruit combined adds up to 65 grams of carbohydrates. Fruit consumption is not a standard recommendation for someone suffering the effects of diabetes because it is stated that fruit contains too much sugar. Counting carbohydrates is encouraged, however, bread, gravy, barbeque sauce, pasta, and pizza are considered acceptable carbohydrates to consume by a dietician. Relying on the statement that "A carb is a carb," complicates health because the only consideration when counting carbs is the carbohydrate to glucose conversion. Considerations for the nutritional content, saturated fat, and chemical additives in the carbohydrates are not calculated.

Your body requires carbohydrates in order to function properly. Consuming the majority of your carbohydrates as fresh, raw fruits provides ultimate nutrition and energy in a delicious, natural package.

4

Cholesterol, Fats, and Oils

Fats and oils (liquid fats) are essential for good health. The body cannot make fats on its own. Eating good sources of fats helps the body absorb vitamins A, D, and E, and enhances the functions of the heart, liver, and nervous systems. Fats and oils contribute to a healthy metabolism and healthy skin, hair, and nails.

A list of foods containing healthy fats and oils include:

- Wild-caught fatty fish such as salmon, albacore tuna, herring, sardines and mackerel (eat limited mackerel due to high mercury content)
- Organic coconuts and coconut oil
- Organic olives and olive oil
- Raw, organic almonds, cashews, hazelnuts, pecans, pistachios, and walnuts
- Organic avocadoes
- Organic eggs
- Organic dark chocolate and cacao
- Organic peanuts and peanut butter
- Organic chia seeds, flax seeds, and sunflower seeds

Healthy fats and oils can help lower LDL cholesterol levels, enhance metabolism, and provide natural sources of Omega-3 for healthy heart function.

Monounsaturated fats are found in liquid plant fats such as olive oil, peanut oil, and safflower oil. Almonds, cashews, pecans, and macadamia nuts offer a great source of monounsaturated fats. Monounsaturated fats help lower LDL cholesterol levels, reduce the risk of disease and cancers, and help cells renew themselves.

Polyunsaturated fats assist with brain function, cardiovascular health, help lower triglyceride cholesterol levels, and lessens the possibility of depression. Some of the healthiest sources for this good type of fat are wild-caught salmon, albacore tuna, organic walnuts, organic flax seeds, and organic oils of safflower, sunflower and corn.

Saturated fats are present in beef, pork, poultry, cheese, milk, yogurts, butter, sour cream, and cream cheese. Saturated fats are a major point of confusion and debate. The following information will help you to eliminate any confusion about the controversial debate as to whether or not saturated fats are good for you. Saturated fats are not all the same. Some are good for you and some are very bad for you. It depends upon the source of the saturated fats.

Consuming wild-caught salmon provides a limited amount of saturated fat in a natural, wholesome source along with good fats—monounsaturated and polyunsaturated fats. Olives are an excellent example of monounsaturated fats, polyunsaturated fats, and a small amount of saturated fats nestled together in a great little natural package.

In comparison, the high amount of saturated fats in a double cheeseburger and french fries are accompanied by harmful trans fats and synthetic components. These saturated fats are excessive and are not naturally provided in conjunction with good fats.

The subject of whether or not saturated fats are healthy does not exist in my mind as a reasonable debate. Monounsaturated fats and polyunsaturated fats are essential for great health and when they are accompanied by a small amount of saturated fats in the same food, it would be nature's way of providing that fat for a purpose.

Saturated fat is not the culprit for disease. Consuming large quantities of saturated fats from unsavory food sources is the culprit. There is a difference between a wholesome natural source of saturated fats and a man-made or man-altered food source.

Wild-caught salmon comes from a river. Almonds and coconuts come from a tree. Seeds come from plants. French fries come from a deep fryer. The answer to the saturated fat debate and if it is good for you or not is easy: if it is in its natural form, the saturated fat is good for you. If it is not in its natural form, the saturated fat is bad for you.

Trans fats occur naturally in meat and milk products in minimal quantities. The majority of all consumed trans fats are synthetic and can be identified as anything containing hydrogenated or partially hydrogenated oils of any kind: vegetable, corn, soy or canola. All foods made with shortening, stick margarine, and lard contain trans fats. Trans fats are extremely dangerous to your good health. They exist in nearly every cooked or fried fast food product, prepackaged baked goods, salty snacks, store-made bakery items, and other artificial foods. Daily consumption of these products on a regular basis prompts heart disease, stroke, diabetes, and cancer.

Cholesterol is a unique and misunderstood story. Since your 10,000-year-old machine was designed as a vegetarian, the body manufactures cholesterol through a biochemical process. Consuming large amounts of cholesterol-laden meats wreaks havoc on the cardiovascular system, the liver, and functions of the brain. Healthy cholesterol ingestion is necessary for bile production in the liver, production of sex hormones, and for cellular and tissue formation. Good cholesterol helps protect your heart and enhances brain function.

Cholesterol, and its different classifications, is somewhat confusing and difficult to comprehend. Your body needs cholesterol in order to perform various functions and *your body creates its own cholesterol.* So here is an easy way to understand this complicated, very important, function of the body. Let's look at the players in the game of cholesterol.

- Good cholesterol is referred to as HDL (High-Density Lipoprotein).
- Bad cholesterol is called LDL (Low-Density Lipoprotein).

Using the analogy of cleaning a chimney, I will explain the pitfalls and heroics of cholesterol. When using a wood stove, the process of burning the wood can create soot in the chimney. If the wood has been dried for the appropriate amount of time and does not contain a lot of sap, then the wood burns cleaner and less soot accumulates in the chimney.

Good wood = less soot in the chimney
Good cholesterol = less build-up in the arteries

Sappy wood = more soot in the chimney
Bad cholesterol = more build-up in the arteries

When you consume a food that contains high amounts of bad cholesterol (LDL), plaque builds up in the arteries. *What most people do not understand is that the good cholesterol (HDL) acts like a chimney sweeper and cleans out the bad cholesterol.* By limiting the amount of LDL and consuming higher amounts of HDL, you can clean out your arteries naturally before disaster strikes.

A chimney needs cleaned out each year before the next heating season begins in order to eliminate the possibility of a chimney fire. Your arteries need cleaned out on a regular basis to eliminate the potential of a heart attack or stroke. *The heroic feat of HDL cholesterol is that it carries the LDL cholesterol out of your arteries, through your blood and into the liver so it can prepare the LDL cholesterol for disposal.*

Your incredible human body is designed to do amazing functions. It can even completely reverse LDL cholesterol issues when you provide the nutritional foundation for the HDL cholesterol to do its job. Understanding the role of cholesterol within the body can help you understand your health situation and how to make better dietary choices.

Where do your favorite foods rank on the following cholesterol chart?

Increases HDL (Good)

Fresh, Raw Fruits/Vegetables		Salmon	Olives
Albacore Tuna	Hazelnuts	Sardines	Garlic
Raw Cacao	Avocados	Green Tea	Beans
Almonds	Black Tea	Walnuts	Prunes
Flax Seed	Chia Seed	Brown Rice	Alfalfa
Wild Rice	Red wine	Legumes	Ginger
Spirulina	Artichoke	Brazil Nuts	Bran

Increases LDL (Bad)

Partially Hydrogenated Vegetable Oil

Red Meat	Fast Food	Caviar	Bacon
Egg Yolks	Sausage	Hot Dogs	Crackers
Salty Snacks	Palm Oil	Deli Meats	Pizza
Shortening/Lard	Organ Meats	Butter	Tacos
Salad Dressing	Mayonnaise	Muffins	Cheese
Non-dairy Creamer	Ice Cream	Pastrami	Cakes
All Fried Foods	Crab	Lobster	Pork

In addition, there are two other cholesterol classifications: triglycerides and Lp(a) cholesterol.

Triglycerides

Triglycerides are used to store energy from excess carbohydrate consumption. Elevated triglycerides can be the result of high LDL/low HDL consumption, alcoholism, smoking, vaping, and other toxic lifestyles.

Lp(a) Cholesterol

Lp(a) is a derivative of LDL (bad) cholesterol and adversely effects your arteries.

As with any element of your health, balance is the key. Understanding cholesterol's role in your body makes you an informed consumer; but more importantly, provides you with an education to establish better eating habits that will ultimately transform into better health.

5

Minerals

Minerals are required for the proper function of the nervous system, development of teeth and bones, support of the immune system, tissue growth and repair, healthy functionality of enzymes and muscle contraction and release.

Minerals must be consumed. Your body does not create them. They are distinguished between Essential, Trace, and Very Trace mineral categories. Minerals contribute an extraordinary role in operating your body's many functions. The functions of minerals are so vast, listing their complete role and their contribution to every function would require writing an entire book dedicated to their service to the human body. The following list is a limited overview of the benefits minerals provide.

Essential Minerals

- ***Calcium*** - development of strong bones and teeth, steady heart rhythms, healthy nerve functions, and muscle contractions; an electrolyte. Found in collard greens, broccoli, kale, figs, oranges, and many other fruits and vegetables.
- ***Chloride*** - production and balance of stomach acids and other fluids. Found in table salt, sea salt, celery, olives, tomatoes and lettuce, just to name a few.
- ***Magnesium*** - protein production/absorption, muscle contraction and release, immune function, nervous system conductivity. Found in cacao, raw nuts, seeds, dark leafy greens, avocadoes, fish, and many other natural sources.

- ***Phosphorus*** - healthy cell function and production. Found in nuts, corn, broccoli, whole wheat, poultry and garlic.
- ***Potassium*** - blood flow, muscle function and nerve transmission. Found in bananas, beet tops, prunes, baked white and sweet potatoes, and fish.
- ***Sodium*** - fluid balance, muscle function, and nerve transmission. Found in natural salt, celery, carrots, egg yolks, kale, red cabbage, and asparagus, for example.
- ***Sulphur*** - present in six amino acids in your body, assists with protein synthesis, enzyme reactions, formation of collagen, aids all cell activity, third most abundant mineral based on percentage of body weight. Found in a variety of green vegetables, nuts, beans, poultry, and fish.[1]

Trace Minerals

- ***Chromium*** - Helps to regulate glucose levels and metabolism. Found in broccoli, oats, tomatoes, mushrooms, seafood, romaine lettuce, green beans, etc.
- ***Copper*** - Required to metabolize iron. Found in cacao, sunflower seeds, mushrooms, lentils, almonds, blackstrap molasses, etc.
- ***Fluoride*** - Helps fortify bones and teeth. Found in oregano oil, wine, grape juice, black tea, dill pickles, olive oil, spinach, myrrh, etc.
- ***Iodine*** - Required for proper thyroid function. Found in kelp, cranberries, wakame, wild-caught salmon, shrimp, scallops, eggs, etc.
- ***Iron*** - Required for red blood cells to carry oxygen (very essential trace mineral). Found in cacao, dark leafy greens, eggs, grapes, peaches, legumes, beef, and poultry.
- ***Manganese*** - Helps control sugar levels, metabolism, thyroid and brain function. Found in raw nuts and seeds, green tea, berries, pineapple, wild-caught seafood, dark leafy greens, legumes, etc.

- ***Molybdenum*** - Catalyst for enzymes, facilitates the breakdown of amino acids.[2] Found in raw nuts, legumes, grains, eggs, soy sauce, cottage cheese, to name a few.
- ***Selenium*** - Antioxidant, supports immune, heart, thyroid and brain function. Found in raw nuts, garlic, shiitake mushrooms, raisins, wild-caught shellfish, chia seeds, etc.
- ***Zinc*** - Immune system, cell regeneration, sperm production and sexual function. Found in cacao, spinach, wild-caught shellfish, flax and pumpkin seeds, garlic, eggs, etc.

Very Trace Minerals

- ***Nickel*** - Vital to metabolism.[3] Found in cacao, raw nuts, mushrooms, variety of vegetables, oysters, barley, legumes, etc.
- ***Vanadium*** - Regulates metabolic function. Found in mushrooms, garlic, black pepper, wild-caught shellfish, beer, wine, grains, green beans, corn, and olive oil, for example.
- ***Cobalt*** - Helps create neurotransmitters and form amino acids. Found in beef, poultry, clams, dark leafy greens, milk, oysters, etc.
- ***Silicon*** - Helps utilize vitamin D, joint flexibility, fortifies hair, nails and skin. Found in whole grains, raisins, green beans, alkaline drinking water, raw nuts, etc.

Mineral deficiencies can cause serious health conditions. Lack of or low consumption of selenium, chromium, and/or iodine can significantly impair thyroid function. Lack of or low consumption of potassium and/or sodium can lead to severe leg cramps, heart arrhythmia, and possibly death. Mineral deficiency is also associated with memory loss, fatigue, and metabolic disorders. These are a few examples. Eating a wide variety of fresh fruits and vegetables, raw nuts, and seeds helps supply the needed minerals for a healthy, highly functioning body.

6

Vitamins

Vitamins are nutrients required for your body to function properly. There are two classifications of vitamins: *fat-soluble and water-soluble.* Fat-soluble vitamins are absorbed through lipid fats in your body then stored in fat cells and your liver. Water-soluble vitamins absorb quickly and the excess is normally eliminated from your body through urination.

Fat-Soluble Vitamins

- ***Vitamin A*** is needed for healthy skin, cell growth, vision, immune function, and protein formation. Orange and red fruits and vegetables and dark green vegetables provide good sources of vitamin A.
- ***Vitamin D*** is essential for strong bones and teeth, liver and muscle function, and to fortify a healthy immune system. When direct sunlight is on the skin, the body can manufacture its own vitamin D. Thirty minutes in the sun, without sunscreen, can provide approximately 10,000-20,000IU of vitamin D. Food sources of vitamin D include Sockeye salmon, albacore tuna, shiitake mushrooms, and eggs.
- ***Vitamin E*** is an antioxidant that helps protect cells from oxidative stress (free radicals). It supports the immune system, cardiovascular and brain health, and serves as a general whole-body health aid. Good natural sources of this vitamin can be found in fatty fish, nuts (almonds, Brazil nuts, and hazelnuts), sunflower seeds, and spirulina.

- ***Vitamin K*** can be made within the body by certain bacteria living in the intestinal tract. It is essential to help your blood coagulate (clot) when you are cut or injured. Natural sources are green tea, spinach and kale.

Fat-soluble vitamins can be stored in the body for long periods. They are stored mostly in the fatty tissue and in the liver. Ingesting good HDL fat helps the body store and utilize fat-soluble vitamins.

Water-Soluble Vitamins

- ***Vitamin B*** includes B1 (thiamine), B2 (riboflavin), B3 (niacin), B5 (pantothenic acid), B6 (pyridoxine), B7 (biotin), B9 (folic acid), and B12 (cobalamin). This variety of B vitamins is required for nervous system function, manufacturing red blood cells, protein metabolism and healthy skin. B vitamins also help to convert carbohydrates into energy. B12 is only found in meat, fish, seafood, poultry and eggs. It is not found in plants. Whole grains, legumes, leafy greens, nuts and fruits can provide adequate sources of the remaining B vitamins.
- ***Vitamin C*** (ascorbic acid) is an antioxidant required for a strong immune system, building connective tissue, fortifying blood vessels, and contributing to protein metabolism. Natural sources of vitamin C can be found in citrus fruits, dark leafy greens, strawberries, cherries, bell peppers, and broccoli, to name a few.

Healthy sources of water-soluble vitamins must be consumed daily because they are not stored in the body.

The easiest way to evaluate the nutrient levels in your body is through a series of blood tests. You will need a copy of the blood test in order to properly assess these levels for your age. There is a very good reason you should not allow a "normal" reading of your blood test to be acceptable to you. For example, the range for potassium is 3.5-5.1 mmol/L. A blood test provides every age with the same "normal" reading. When the results of the blood tests are within the acceptable range, regardless of age, the results are considered to be normal and acceptable.

In high school, the grading scale was 60-100 percent. If you received a 95 to 100, it was an A+, but a 64 percent was a failing grade. A 64 percent was still within the 60-100 percent range, but was not good enough to receive a passing grade in the class. When reading your blood test, apply the same grading scale principle. Using potassium as an example, a 25-year-old, seemingly healthy male would not remain very healthy for long if his blood test results revealed 3.7 mmol/L. He would be within the acceptable range (3.5-5.1 mmol/L), but this number would be very low for his age.

Relating this to the high school grading scale, this young man receives an F, a failing grade. If a 92-year-old man had the same results, it may be understandable considering his age, activity level, and the requirements of his aging body to process and maintain a higher level of potassium. Potassium plays such an important role in the body, that having such a low, yet normal blood level result for a very active 25-year-old, can be the reason for muscle cramps, digestion issues, fatigue, irregular heartbeat, ulcerative colitis, Crohn's disease, low bone density, and possible stroke during excessive workouts.

Lack of appropriate vitamin intake directly correlates to a weakened immune system. Without a strong immune system, defense against oxidative damage becomes limited and you are more susceptible to disease. Ensure you are receiving appropriate vitamin levels by consuming a variety of fresh, raw organic fruits and vegetables.

Many bad habits have been established that inhibit great health: stress, lacking a proper night's sleep, working more than forty hours a week, eating junk that we refer to as food, and neglecting a healthy diet and exercise program. A barrage of advertisements for medications on television make it easy to perceive that abusing the body and neglecting nutrition can be fixed with a pill. It cannot. A diseased body absolutely cannot be fixed or cured with a pill. The body demands that the rules designed by nature for a healthy body cannot be substituted with shortcuts.

"Nutrition is the major factor being neglected and ignored as a fundamental necessity for a healthy human existence."
– DK Guyer, PhD

I conducted a small-scale survey of fifty people at two different locations to determine how much people knew about nutrition. Knowing that a conversation about nutrition would not be an interesting subject, I approached it in this manner. Standing outside a pet store, I asked the following questions:

"Do you know the nutritional requirements for your pet to stay healthy?" One hundred percent answered "Yes" or "Yes, I think so."

"Do you know the nutritional requirements for you to stay healthy?" One hundred percent answered with laughter. Then I received these responses:

"I know I could do a better job." – 16 people
"I know what I should be doing. I just don't do it." – 11 people
"I'm too lazy to cook the right things." – 7 people
"I don't like vegetables." – 6 people
"I don't eat right, but I take vitamins." – 6 people
"I'm just a meat and potatoes person." – 1 person
"I'm going to start eating healthy next week. – 1 person
"I eat bacon for protein. That's healthy, right?" – 1 person
"I'm 81. Still driving. Still walking. Must be doing something right." – 1 person

At the end of each response, I offered a thank you for their time and stated in a very nice way that it was extremely generous of the person to take better care of their pet than themselves. They all laughed and agreed. Everyone was kind and friendly.

The only person I did not offer that response to was the 81-year-old man. He looked much younger than what I pictured an 81-year-old man to appear, so I asked him to share his secret. He responded, "I grow my own food so no corporation can ruin it." He then hurried off.

The second survey was at an automotive garage. "Do you know the requirements for your car to be properly maintained?" One hundred percent answered "Yes" or "I'm pretty sure I do."

"Do you know the nutritional requirements for you to stay healthy?" Ten percent answered with laughter. Then I received these responses:

"Not really." – 15 people
"No." – 11 people
"Yes." or "Yep." – 10 people
"Don't really care." – 8 people
"I get a blood test every 3 months to make sure my meds aren't killing me." – 1 person
"I didn't come with a manual." – 1 person
"I don't know the particulars, but try to eat healthy." – 1 person (while drinking a diet soda)
"I take vitamins." – 1 person
"I just eat what I want." – 1 person
"I guess so. I'm still here." – 1 person (age 42)

At the end of each response, I offered a thank you for their time and stated in a very nice way that it was extremely generous of the person to take better care of their car than themselves. This crowd was not as upbeat and friendly as the participants at the pet store. Some laughed. Some ignored me. Most of the people I spoke with appeared unhappy to be there and viewed my survey as annoying. I guess if you have to have your car fixed, it truly impacts your attitude.

The bottom line is that most people have the same approach to health—ignore it and the warning signs until there is a crisis and then rely on a pill to fix it.

The biggest complaint about embracing a diet designed to provide extraordinary health is being hungry all the time, the probability of having diarrhea, and a perceived higher cost at the grocery store. These are serious concerns to those who wish to change to a healthier diet and fret about the unknown. Let's address these concerns.

Objections to Eating a Healthy Diet

Causes Hunger

When you provide your body with nutrition, you are not always hungry. Yes. Oh, heavens, yes! You will eat less! Here is the proof. When you go to a buffet and eat until you are stuffed to the point of unbuckling your pants or loosening your belt, how is it then that you can be hungry again within four hours? You have already consumed more food than a household of four people in Japan, China, Greece, and Italy eats in one day. Yet, you are hungry. Yes, you absolutely are hungry. Your body wants nutrients! It is begging you for nutrients!

You just ate a buffet plate, or second plate, full of cooked, nutrient-deprived, sodium-filled, contaminated, synthetic, non-digestible, non-usable garbage. So the body is not asking for food to fill the stomach, you feel hungry after eating all that junk because your body is asking for nutrition. Not just a belly full of stuff.

As a statistic, Americans are overfed, undernourished, diseased, and obese. Can you imagine why? People eat and eat and mistake the body's request for nutrition as a need for foodstuff and as a result, consume massive amounts of unusable contents. This type of eating experience symbolizes how little many Americans respect their health and longevity.

Not only is the buffet a danger zone for foodstuffs of little or no nutritional value, the items are made with higher fat and sodium content than most anything you would cook for yourself at home. The first danger is overeating. The second danger is consuming more fat and sodium in one meal than the body should consume in one month! The third danger zone is the price. Eating at a buffet costs on average $12-$19 per person. Following the suggested diet options in this book, you will eat less than $7-$8 for the entire day while satiating your body with much needed nutrients, not feeling hungry, improving your health and feeling the best you've ever felt. When discussing food costs one on one with individuals concerned that they cannot afford fresh fruits and vegetables or eat organic foods, we get out the shopping receipts or start going through the cupboards and refrigerator, because it is not a fact. Most grocery lists contain items that *make* you hungry. They are unneeded, toxic, synthetic products with a high price tag and contain nothing of nutritional value.

When you purchase products that provide full nutrition, you are not hungry. When your belly rumbles and you interpret it as hunger, and then you consume synthetic products with no nutrition, your body responds by continually expressing hunger. Eating products with nutrients not only suppresses the continuous need to consume foodstuffs, but it provides nutrition that helps every function within your body. You eat less. You lose weight. You spend less money on food. You spend less time in the kitchen. You spend less energy cooking and cleaning because you are eating more raw fruits and vegetables. You have little or no need for purchasing over-the-counter medicines and antacids. You will have the money you saved on the grocery bill, visits to the doctor, and eating out to purchase a new wardrobe to fit your new, lean healthy body.

"Let us focus on the most important issues:
Eat primarily whole raw natural foods. Avoid the real killers—tobacco, alcohol, drugs, coffee, refined sugar, salt, environmental pollutants, high-protein diets, and, for that matter overeating in general."
–Dr. Ralph Cinque, 1985

Causes Diarrhea

People experience diarrhea every day of the week, but it is rarely because they are adopting a healthier food consumption regimen. The number one reason for not eating fresh fruits and vegetables daily is the perceived notion that it will cause diarrhea. It is neither the price tag nor the dislike of fresh fruits and vegetables. It is merely the lack of education.

People experience diarrhea after eating at certain Chinese restaurants because the majority of the food contains MSG (monosodium glutamate). The body treats MSG as poison, thus producing diarrhea. The same response is true when consuming too much alcohol. The body's natural defense is to expel the toxins.

Shopping list of an average American:

Product	*Dangers*
Hot dogs	Listed as carcinogenic by WHO
Bacon	Listed as carcinogenic by WHO
Cereal	GMO grains, artificial flavors and preservatives
Soda	Artificial flavors, sugars
Cookies	GMO grains, artificial flavors, sugars, preservatives
Deli meat	Highly contaminated with chemicals, high sodium
Bread	Potassium Bromate, Yeast, GMO flour, additives
Ice Cream	Chemicals, contaminated milk, yeast extract
Chicken	Steroids, antibiotics, hormones, chemicals
Barbeque sauce	Chemicals, sugar, sodium
Potatoes	Chemicals, starch
Potato chips	High in Sodium, chemicals, trans fats
Can soup	High in Sodium, chemicals, trans fats
Can vegetables	High in Sodium, chemicals, little to no nutrition
Pasta	GMO grains, chemicals, preservatives
Spaghetti sauce	Chemicals, sugar, sodium
Eggs	Steroids, antibiotics, hormones, chemicals
Cheese	Steroids, antibiotics, hormones, chemicals
Fruit Juice	Artificial flavors, colors, sugar, preservatives
Box mac/cheese	GMO grains, artificial flavors, colors, sodium, preservatives
Box meals	GMO grains, artificial flavors, colors, sodium, preservatives
Hamburger in tube	Known as pink slime. That should say it all.
Hamburger buns	Potassium bromate, sodium, preservatives
Hot dog buns	Potassium bromate, sodium, preservatives
Fish sticks	Farm raised fish, sodium, preservatives, chemicals
Frozen pizza	Sodium, yeast extract, preservatives, synthetic toppings
Milk	Steroids, antibiotics, hormones, chemicals
Coffee	Chemically processed
Coffee creamer	Chemicals
Sugar	Chemicals
Flour	GMO grains, chemicals
Applesauce	Sugar, preservatives, pesticides
Enhanced water	Aspartame, artificial flavor
Crackers	GMO grains, artificial flavors, colors, sodium, preservatives
Cream cheese	Steroids, antibiotics, hormones, chemicals
Pancake mix	GMO grains, artificial flavors, colors, sodium, preservatives
Syrup	High fructose corn syrup, artificial flavors, colors, sodium
Ibuprofen	Synthetic inactive ingredients
Antacid	Calcium carbonate, magnesium hydroxide, artificial color

Compare that list to the healthy shopping list that follows:

Organic spring mix salad greens
Organic nuts
Organic bananas
Organic carrots
Organic celery
Organic green pepper
Organic cucumber
Organic tomatoes
Organic vegetable or chicken broth
Organic apples
Organic eggs
Organic milk
Organic cereal
Organic chicken
Organic tea or coffee
Organic tortilla chips
Organic flour
Organic olives
Organic berries
Organic sweet potatoes
Organic raisins
Organic beets
Organic cottage cheese
Organic beets
Wild-caught salmon

Have you ever heard or witnessed any of these following situations?

- An overweight person orders a double cheeseburger, french fries, an ice cream sundae, and a diet soda and then complains that she cannot lose weight.
- A belligerent person yells at the waitress because every time he eats there, he gets a bad case of heartburn and indigestion—after eating an oversized pulled pork sandwich, onion rings, mozzarella sticks with red sauce, and a huge soda.
- At a tailgate party, someone loudly announces that he has to have an antacid before he can eat another bite and goes

through the parking lot to find someone who will generously donate the needed antacid so he can eat his fourth hamburger and start his second six-pack of beer.

- A mother disgustingly tells the other parents at the Parent Teacher meeting that her child refuses to eat anything but macaroni and cheese or french fries. Then proceeds to blame the teachers for bullying her child because he will not pay attention or stay in his seat.
- A coach encourages his team to eat an extra-large meal for dinner and a big breakfast in the morning because they have an important game tomorrow. They will need their strength, he adds. At half time, he admonishes their performance because they are sluggish.

People rarely equate fatigue, sluggish athletic performance or focus with their eating habits. And rarely can anyone tell you how much sodium, fat, calories, or cholesterol they have consumed in a day. Daily nutrition is not a standard habit. The true facts about nutrition and how your body operates is not common knowledge.

If you get heartburn or indigestion after eating something, please quit eating it, or at least try chewing it up before you swallow it. Your body is telling you it cannot handle the stuff you are putting in your stomach. After four hamburgers and a six-pack of beer in a short period of time, you most likely are going to feel awful.

After eating an extra-large dinner and a big breakfast before a game, you will feel sluggish. Your body is using energy to digest all that food instead of fueling your body. We have all witnessed people feeling badly after abusing their body during a party or a night out drinking or overeating, but their bad habits do not cease. Children with behavioral problems are nearly always nutrient deficient.

We have become complacent as a society when it comes to nutrition and paying attention to what our bodies are telling us. Rather than analyze what we are doing to contribute to the health situation, it becomes commonplace to blame someone or something else.

This is an account of an actual conversation. A man is telling me of all his horrific health issues. We will call him Mike.

Then I ask, "When was the last time you ate fresh fruits and vegetables, Mike?"

His response, "I can't eat that stuff. It gives me diarrhea."

"You only get diarrhea when you eat fruits and vegetables?" I asked politely with a smile.

He says, "Sometimes. If I drink too much on Friday night or order Chinese take-out, I get diarrhea." Then he smiled and lowered his head.

I respond, "So you have had diarrhea before and it has nothing to do with eating fresh fruits and vegetables. Mike, that's not a good excuse. What's the real reason?" and then I paused. "Maybe you just don't like fruits and vegetables?"

He says, "Vegetables are for wimps. I need REAL food!" clenching his fists and arm muscles like a power lifter.

What is a person to say to that answer?!

"If you truly want to be well and start feeling better, you need to get some nutrition. Eating fresh organic fruits and vegetables is the easiest way to do that. If that isn't something you are willing to try, I'm very limited in options that can help you. I eat fresh fruits and vegetables every day. Maybe you are just a special breed of human who doesn't need nutrition; you can just eat junk food to survive." I said in a light-hearted, half laughing way.

He says, "You call this surviving? I'm on twelve different prescriptions and feel like hell every day!"

"Mike, no one is forcing you to buy this stuff," as I reach in the cart to hold up a package of flavored pretzels. "Your cart is full of junk food. Not only are you paying the consequences of feeling bad, you are also paying a huge price tag at the checkout to voluntarily make yourself sick," I said.

"You really believe that hoopla that fruits and vegetables are important?" he responded.

"Absolutely," I said. "Your body needs vitamins, minerals, water, and food made in nature to be healthy. It is not heredity that contributes to your health issues, it's nutrition. You are a human being and a very kind one. You are not a garbage can," I added.

He lowered his head and said, "My grandmother is ninety-four years old. My mother is seventy-five years old and she doesn't take any medicine. I know I come from great genes. That's why I can't understand why I have all these diseases that people inherit from their family."

"Disease is rarely inherited. It is earned. By abusing your body, you welcome disease. If you don't provide it with nutrition, how is it supposed to function properly?" I responded.

"It sounds like you're telling me I have to give up my favorite foods. I'm not sure I can do that," he said knowing that his argument held no validity.

"It is your choice if you want to change your eating habits. No one is forcing you to eat fast food. No one admonishes you for not consuming water. No one will feel the pain of your declining health, but you. It is one hundred percent your choice what you eat. What was your favorite fruit as a kid?" I asked.

"Peaches. I love peaches. I would steal them from the orchard near our house every chance I got. Apples, too. I used to eat fruit at home. Fruit pies. Fresh fruit on my cereal. Fruit on my pancakes. Fruit in my lunch at school," he responded with a happy tone in his voice. His tone then changed back to being concerned.

"I guess that is why mom and grandma are still so healthy. They eat fresh fruit every day. I live alone and don't have much time to shop. I guess I need to change that a bit. Do you think I could get off some of these meds if I eat fruit and vegetables?" he asked sheepishly.

"Giving your body real nutrition can help eliminate the symptoms of all your conditions. If you eat properly this Tuesday but then eat junk food for the next week, it is not going to get you off your meds. You have to be consistent and let your doctor know you are changing your eating habits and want to get off the medications. We are Americans and this is the land of the free. It is your choice every single day what you purchase and what you ingest as food. You are in control of your health," I said.

"You might be on to something. I think I'll take a stab at adding some fruits and vegetables. I can't argue with the Garden of Eden in the Bible. God put great stuff on this earth. I just like the taste of fried stuff. Chicken and pizza and Mexican and Chinese and fried potatoes and gravy. I guess that stuff isn't good for you after all. Can you help me? I know I'm a losing cause. But is there any way you can help me?" he asked.

"I can help get you started on a better diet and a healthier lifestyle," I said.

"I have to do something. I can barely make it to work I feel so bad," he uttered.

"I've seen you in action when you make up your mind to do something. You can do this, Mike. I will tell you what I eat and how to get started," I said cheerfully.

This conversation occurred in a grocery store. Mike lived alone. We had met through a community service project. He was passionate about helping others. His grocery cart was filled with diet soda, frozen dinners, salty snacks, ice cream products, and candy. He was obese, red-faced, and ill. Viewing my cart, he commented on the price I must be paying. With our cell phone calculators, we added the cost of the items. His cart exceeded mine by $80 and some change. I was buying for three. He was buying for himself.

After three months, he was off all his prescription medications. All of them! He had lost more than 80 pounds in three months and felt, in his words, "Great." With the savings from buying real food and being off prescription medications, he hired someone to prepare his evening meals and wash and cut his fresh fruits and vegetables and put them in either containers or lunch bags for his at-work meals. He saved enough money in three months changing his eating habits and getting off prescription medications, not only to afford paying someone $175 a week to help with food preparation, but to save enough money for a vacation! He thanked me for everything I did.

I did not do the work. He did. He just needed someone to walk him through the steps and prove that it would work even though his mother and grandmother practiced the essentials I described to him.

Knowledge is a powerful thing. Mike is a very intelligent and successful man, but he truly did not know that the way he was eating was destroying his health. He thought that if it was on the grocery store shelf, it couldn't be *that* bad for him. Many people share the same thoughts as Mike. They purchase foods they like and that are quick and easy to prepare.

The mother whose child eats french fries and macaroni and cheese probably is not aware of the health complications waiting to surface due to her child's lack of nutrition. The coach who thinks he is helping his team by telling them to eat an extra-large dinner and big breakfast truly does not know the resulting impaired athletic performance of such a statement.

People go through stages. They eat whatever they can afford to eat during their low-cost first years away from home. Once they get better jobs and a stable income, the choice remains: buy quality food and eat at home or spend it on higher priced processed foods and eating out. This new choice determines their health.

Purchasing organic produce helps eliminate some of the diarrhea issue. Non-organic produce contains pesticide residue. Even when the produce is washed, the pesticides have already made their way inside the produce by penetrating the outer surface. One function of the body is to eliminate toxic material as quickly as possible to preserve the life and health of its cells and tissue. Eating pesticide-laden produce can evoke diarrhea. So there is some truth to getting diarrhea from eating non-organic fresh fruits and vegetables.

The following is a list of fruits and vegetables that contain higher amounts of chemical contamination. They are the most heavily sprayed crops and the list is referred to as the "Dirty Dozen":

1. Apples
2. Peaches
3. Nectarines
4. Strawberries
5. Grapes
6. Celery
7. Spinach
8. Sweet bell peppers
9. Cucumbers
10. Cherry tomatoes
11. Snap peas (imported)
12. Potatoes

The human body operates on nutrition. There is no substitute. Vitamins and minerals are essential for good health. Diarrhea is not a reason for neglecting organic fresh fruits and vegetables, it is just an excuse.

There is hope. You can redesign your health, your future happy, healthy existence by changing your eating habits.

7

Water Consumption

Everyone knows that water is essential for life. Human existence has either thrived or perished over the centuries depending on access to pure water for consumption. The body can last a few weeks without ingesting food; but without water, life cannot survive for very long. Absolutely every single cell in the body requires water for proper function. Every time you swallow, speak, blink, move, laugh, chew, walk, run, sit, sleep, breath, and think, your body requires water for that to happen. Your heart, spine, digestive system, nerves, muscles, bones, skin, eyes, brain, blood vessels, hair, and tendons require water to operate or grow. The reason I am listing these functions is that every person suffers from lack of water at some point in their lives.

Here is the water content of:

Blood	92%
Brain	75%
Muscles	70% - 75%
Bones	20% - 25% (dependent on age; younger bones contain more water)

Nearly every person has experienced some of the effects of dehydration: headache, dizziness, muscle cramps, and fatigue. Lack of water presents many different symptoms because it is required for every function of the body. The reason so many people suffer the effects of dehydration is twofold.

First, they consume coffee, ready-to-drink teas, energy drinks, juices, alcoholic beverages, or soda instead of water. These beverages contain chemicals and sugars, producing a diuretic effect that removes water from the body. Second, they consume massive amounts of dry, synthetic foods that further diminish the body's water content.

Organic, fresh, raw fruits, and vegetables contain water. It is easy to recognize how nourishing and hydrating a fresh, juicy peach is to the body compared to a dry, salty snack.

Percentage of water content in fruits and vegetables:[1]

Strawberry	92%	Cucumber	96%
Watermelon	92%	Lettuce, Iceberg	96%
Grapefruit	91%	Celery	95%
Cantaloupe	90%	Radish	95%
Peaches	88%	Zucchini	95%
Cranberry	87%	Tomato	94%
Orange	87%	Cabbage, Green	93%
Pineapple	87%	Cabbage, Red	92%
Raspberry	87%	Cauliflower	92%
Apricot	86%	Eggplant	92%
Blueberry	85%	Peppers, Bell	92%
Plum	85%	Spinach	92%
Apples	84%	Broccoli	91%
Pears	84%	Carrots	87%
Cherries	81%	Green Peas	79%
Grapes	81%	White Potato	79%
Bananas	74%		

Eating fresh fruits and vegetables provides antioxidants, various nutrients, and valuable water content for hydration.

Water consumption rules are not written in stone. Some experts advise using your weight divided in half to calculate the amount of water you should consume. Other experts advise taking your weight and multiplying it by two-thirds to calculate the amount. *These rules can be very dangerous!* Here is the reason why. For a person who has had their thyroid removed and is dependent upon medication to replace that function, this extraordinary amount of water can flush out the medication and reduce the medication's effectiveness. Furthermore, recovering alcoholics and narcotics users may have limited liver and kidney function, and consuming large amounts of water instead of gradually increasing water intake can cause an array of health complications due to the inability of the compromised organs to operate normally. The average healthy individual could experience heart attack or stroke when consuming excessive water due to severe loss of sodium and electrolytes. The body is a delicate balance of water and sodium.

Electrolytes are minerals (sodium, potassium, chloride, calcium, magnesium, bicarbonate, and hydrogen phosphate) that carry an electrical charge. They are required for full functionality of the brain, heart, nervous system, muscles, and so much more. Dividing your weight in half and consuming that amount of water without regard to electrolyte loss and resupply is very dangerous.

This is my recommendation. Drink 6 to 8 ounces of water first thing in the morning before you begin getting ready for your day. Eat fresh fruits for breakfast that contain at least 70 percent water. You will begin your day hydrated. Snack on fresh fruit if you are hungry before lunch time. Drink 8 ounces of water 30 to 45 minutes before lunch. Eat a large fresh salad with a variety of high water content vegetables and fruits. Drink 8 ounces of water mid-afternoon and another 8 ounces 30 to 45 minutes before dinner. Drink 6 to 8 ounces of water two hours before bedtime. This practice will establish a habit that will help keep you hydrated but you are not limited, specifically, to this amount of water. Other factors such as physical activity, heat index, your age, and health conditions, along with how much or little you perspire contribute to whether you need more water intake.

Monitoring the color and clarity of your first urination of the morning is a determining sign as to whether or not you are consuming appropriate amounts of water. If your urine is not clear or presents an odor, you need to drink more water. Dark or foul odor urine is a clear indicator that you are dehydrated.

The use of synthetic products, tobacco, alcohol, soda, coffee, drug use, and prescription medications contributes to dehydration.

Clear or very next to clear when you urinate after a six to eight-hour sleep period is your goal. If this is not the case, increase your water consumption.

There is a direct correlation between high blood pressure and water consumption. When you drink excessive amounts of water without taking in appropriate amounts of real sodium sources, you endanger your life. The human body requires a delicate balance of real sodium and water. Sodium nitrates contained in processed or packaged foods are not a real source of sodium. They are synthetic. Real sodium comes from sea salt and certain vegetables. When sodium decreases to a very low level, the body shuts down. Everyone needs a minimum of 1,800 to 2,000 mg of sodium daily when drinking five to six 8 ounce glasses of water and experiencing normal mobility. If you ingest a high sodium diet, you will need to drink much more water to stabilize your blood pressure than someone who monitors their sodium intake.

If you are perspiring due to excessive heat and activity, monitor your loss of sodium and water by how much you sweat. When you perspire excessively, you will require more water and more sodium. Both are lost during intense activity and perspiration.

The amount of water your body requires is directly related to your activity level, sodium intake, and fresh fruit and vegetable consumption, not your weight.

Have Your Water Tested

Most water companies offer free water testing. When you are opting to consume more water for better health, you will want to ensure that is it alkaline and free from dangerous contaminants.

The most common objection to drinking water is a strong dislike for the taste. When water is contaminated, it can present an undesirable flavor. Once your water has been tested and the issues are remedied, if you still dislike the taste, try adding a slice of orange, lemon, or lime to add natural flavor. Using organic frozen strawberries, raspberries, or blueberries will add flavor and chill your water at the same time.

Water is the fountain of youth—the fountain of life. I hope you can find a way to enjoy it.

When you learn how to care for your body, better health follows. Even the most dire health conditions can be altered for the better when the body receives the nutriment it requires. Water is an important requirement.

The following is a list from the Environmental Protection Agency[2] for your consideration when judging your water:

Conditions or Nearby Activities	Recommended Test
Recurrent gastro-intestinal illness	Coliform bacteria
Household plumbing contains lead	**pH, lead, copper**
Radon in indoor air or region is radon rich	Radon
Scaly residues, soaps don't lather	**Hardness**
Water softener needed to treat hardness	Manganese, iron
Stained plumbing fixtures, laundry	**iron, copper, manganese**
Objectionable taste or smell	Hydrogen sulfide, corrosion, metals
Water appears cloudy, frothy or colored	**Color, detergents**
Corrosion of pipes, plumbing	Corrosion, pH, lead
Rapid wear of water treatment equipment	**pH, corrosion**
Nearby areas of intensive agriculture	Nitrate, pesticides, coliform bacteria
Coal or other mining operation nearby	**Metals, pH, corrosion**
Gas drilling operation nearby	Chloride, sodium, barium, strontium
Odor of gasoline or fuel oil, and near gas station or buried fuel tanks	**Volatile organic compounds (VOC)**
Dump, junkyard, landfill, factory or dry-cleaning operation nearby	VOC, Total dissolved solids (TDS), pH, sulfate, chloride
Salty taste and seawater, or a heavily salted roadway nearby	**Chloride, TDS, sodium**

8

Where Do Diseases Originate?

Cellular destruction sounds very complicated, but I will demonstrate with examples of how this happens in your body, why it is important for you to understand the process, and how to stop the occurrence and consequential destruction in an easy-to-understand format.

First of all, your body is a healing machine! Given the right nutrition, anything in your body can heal as long as it is still functioning.

A broken arm heals in a cast in six weeks. Just think about that statement for a moment. A bone broken in half is healed back together in forty-two days! The body is an incredible healing machine and you own it.

A thumb smashed with a hammer that loses the fingernail will experience swelling, aching, and in a few days, a brand-new thumb nail begins to grow, the swelling recedes, and the thumb is once again usable.

These examples are to establish in your mind the undeniable proof that your body can heal itself. All of our cells are preprogrammed to adjust to damages and to repair dead or damaged tissue.

If you cut yourself while shaving, you most likely will not run to the hospital emergency room, because you know the bleeding will cease and the cut will heal. This same response occurs inside your body when you ingest toxic materials that destroy your tissues.

Once the body reaches a certain level of toxicity, the cells will start to break down past the point of repair unless immediate changes are made. Smoking two packs of cigarettes a day will cause cellular damage in your mouth, throat, esophagus, lungs, liver, heart, and blood vessels. When you stop smoking and are no longer drawing the toxic material into your body, the cellular damage associated with smoking begins to recover with proper nutrition. By supplying your cells, both healthy and damaged, with needed oxygen, antioxidants, a variety of nutrients, and an appropriate amount of water, your body can begin to remove the damaged and dead cells, restore existing cells, and regenerate healthy new cells.

When you do not stop smoking and continue destroying the cells in every part of your body, the death and destruction of too many cells makes it impossible for regeneration of the cells to occur. You can relate this concept to a simple example—rusting metal on an automobile. When the rust first begins, it can be treated so that the rust does not continue. Aftercare, such as keeping the road salt washed off the automobile during winter and keeping it in a garage to limit exposure to certain weather conditions, can keep the rust issue at bay.

The same response occurs within the body. Your body in a toxic condition is considered to have toxemia. The human body is not designed to tolerate consumption of synthetic materials or highly acidic foods, and over time will become toxic to the point of disease. Cells require an alkaline environment to regenerate and remain healthy. They cannot repair themselves in harsh, or acidic, environments.

Nearly every disease can be halted with appropriate nutrition, suspending the ingestion of toxic materials responsible for the cellular damage, getting enough rest, water, sunlight, and a positive, loving, supportive environment.

Each cell bases its functioning on its pH level. In order to achieve health and maintain it, the body requires a pH level of 7.4. The symbol pH is used to represent the level or degree of acidity or alkalinity of a substance. The acid/alkaline values associated with food are referred to as the PRAL list. PRAL is the abbreviation for Potential Renal Acid Load and was developed by Thomas Remer, PhD and Friedrich Manz, MD. The body requires

80 percent of its daily intake to be alkaline foods and 20 percent to have acidic values to function at its maximum potential. Disease cannot live in an alkalized body.

Because the majority of food produced in the United States of America is processed and/or synthetically modified, the average American has an incredibly acidic daily intake unless a conscious choice is made to ingest alkaline foods. In reviewing your acidic food intake, consider that since the PRAL list was compiled in 1995, this list does not account for the majority of food additives and hormones that exist today.

At the end of the day when you realize that your acidic food consumption numbers are drastically higher than they should be by using this chart, keep in mind that as alarming as those numbers may be to you, this number is actually low in reality. In comparison to what an updated, 2017 version of the PRAL would look like, that highly acidic number that was just tallied would be even higher once it encompassed all the foods containing synthetic additives that did not exist in 1995.

Furthermore, nearly every meal consumed is inadequately combined and impairs proper digestion. So how are any of us still alive? Our cells are incredible and strive to sustain life.

Cells will use every reserve of nutriment in the body to stay alive, which can result in disease. Cells will confiscate calcium and other minerals from the bones in order to operate the organs when calcium is not being ingested. The result of this action is osteoporosis, which it is not a disease. Osteoporosis is the direct result of the lack of nutrition the body is getting and what the body is willing to do out of desperation for the minerals and vitamins it craves.

Another primary example is Crohn's disease. When the intestines are robbed of their nutriment, the result of this action is not a disease but is the result of little or no nutritional content in your food choices.

The following PRAL charts[1] provide information for a variety of highly consumed items. The negative numbers represent alkaline foods. The positive numbers are acidic foods.

PRAL LIST **ACIDIC FOODS**

Meat and Meat Products	
Lean Beef	7.8
Chicken	8.7
Canned, Corned Beef	13.2
Frankfurters	6.7
Liver Sausage	10.6
Lunch Meat	10.2
Lean Pork	7.9
Rump Steak	8.8
Salami	11.6
Turkey Meat	9.9
Veal Fillet	9.0
Sugar and Sweets	
Milk Chocolate	2.4
Cake	3.7
Bread, Flour and Noodles	
Mixed Grain Rye Bread	4.0
Rye Bread	4.1
Mixed Grain Wheat Bread	3.8
Wheat Bread	1.8
White Bread	3.7
Cornflakes	6.0
Rye Crackers	3.3
Egg Noodles	6.4
Oats	10.7
Brown Rice	12.5
White Rice	1.7
Rye Flour	5.9
White Spaghetti	6.5
Whole Grain Spaghetti	7.3
Wheat Flour	8.2
Fats and Oils	
Butter	0.6

Fish	
Cod Fillet	7.1
Haddock	6.8
Herring	7.0
Trout	10.8
Milk, Dairy, Eggs	
Buttermilk	0.5
Low Fat Cheddar	26.4
Gouda Cheese	18.6
Cottage Cheese	8.7
Sour Cream	1.2
Whole Egg	8.2
Egg white	1.1
Egg Yolk	23.4
Hard Cheese	19.2
Ice Cream	0.6
Whole Milk	1.1
Whole Milk Pasteurized	0.7
Parmesan Cheese	34.2
Processed Cheese	28.7
Whole Milk Yogurt w/Fruit	1.2
Whole Milk Yogurt Plain	1.5
Beverages	
Pale Beer	0.9
Coca-Cola	0.4
Legumes	
Lentils	3.5
Peas	1.2
Fruits, Nuts, and Juices	
Peanuts	8.3
Walnuts	6.8

PRAL LIST

ALKALINE FOODS

Sugar and Sweets	
Honey	-0.3
Marmalade	-1.5
White Sugar	-0.1
Vegetables	
Asparagus	-0.4
Broccoli	-1.2
Carrots	-4.9
Cauliflower	-4.0
Celery	-5.2
Chicory	-2.0
Cucumber	-0.8
Eggplant	-3.4
Leeks	-1.8
Lettuce	-2.5
Mushrooms	-1.4
Onions	-1.5
Peppers	-1.4
Potatoes	-4.0
Radishes	-3.7
Spinach	-14.0
Tomato Juice	-2.8
Tomatoes	-3.1
Zucchini	-2.6
Beverages	
Draft Beer	-0.2
Stout Beer	-0.1
White Wine	-1.2
Red Wine	-2.4

Legumes	
Green Beans	-3.1
Fats and Oils	
Margarine	-0.5
Olive Oil	0
Sunflower Oil	0
Fruits, Nuts, and Juices	
Apple Juice	-2.2
Apples	-2.2
Apricots	-4.8
Bananas	-5.5
Black Currants	-6.5
Cherries	-3.6
Grape Juice	-1.0
Hazelnuts	-2.8
Kiwi Fruit	-4.1
Lemon Juice	-2.5
Orange Juice	-2.9
Oranges	-2.7
Peaches	-2.4
Pears	-2.9
Raisins	-21.0
Strawberries	-2.2
Watermelon	-1.9
Beverages	
Cocoa	-0.4
Coffee	-1.4
Mineral water	-1.8
Tea	-0.3

I rearranged the original PRAL list so that all the acidic food values were together and all the alkaline food values were listed together for your convenience.

Using the PRAL list, the most shocking revelation to anyone unfamiliar with this information is that cheese, meat, brown rice, and fish top the chart for acidic foods.

There Is Hope

Occasionally when an alkaline substance is ingested that contains real nutrition, it will help restore the reserves of nutriment. For many people, the day will come when the cells of the body can no longer borrow what is needed to sustain life, and the reserves will be gone completely. This degree of cellular destruction lands these unfortunates in the danger zone. At this point a choice has to made. Should one fight to live or choose to die? Only by achieving the proper pH balance can the body recover to any level. Once the body begins to shut down normal functionality such as urination, food consumption and digestion, mobility, and motor function, at this unfortunate stage, recovery back to any manner of health is foregone.

I have had, on many occasions, spoken with diseased individuals about restoring their health. It amazes me every time I hear an ill person state that giving up cigarettes, hard liquor, bacon, diet soda, and/or cheese to restore their health is not an option. They would rather die than give up their favorite vice. This is an important opportunity I must take to remind all of those with full, loving hearts, that not everyone wants help, has a desire to live full, rich lives, and that, although it is painful, those who do not wish to better themselves cannot be made well. Each person is uniquely their own individual and only they can make the choice that is right for them. If someone chooses to ingest every sort of toxin until their final breath, it is their choice. Love them with an overflowing heart and you have, in fact, done all you can do.

A Chemical Cocktail

In the following example, I will clearly demonstrate how the same toxin can create different diseases.

Pacific Gas and Electric settled a lawsuit filed for the contamination of the drinking water in Hinkley, California. The persons affected by the contaminant, hexavalent chromium, suffered a variety of health complications associated with their levels of exposure.

The point of discussing this lawsuit is to highlight a realization: each affected person displayed different symptoms and different diseases due to their level of contamination and their bodies' nutriment level to combat the toxins. *The hexavalent chromium was the reason for their declining health, but it did not produce the same disease in every individual.*

It is extremely important to understand that just because you have different symptoms than someone else, does not mean the disease was created by different influences. All disease comes from the same thing—too many toxins and not enough nutrition.

Learning about toxic materials and how the body responds to them should shed new light on what you choose to ingest and feed your family. New diseases are erupting at an alarming rate. Often, new and rare forms of cancer, complications in the intestinal tract, and cardiovascular issues are being studied and named. This is not surprising considering that new synthetic food additives are being released into the market as quickly as new diseases are being diagnosed. The correlation is evident. The new forms of toxins in the food supply result in new forms of disease symptoms. When you consider the variety of toxins each individual can consume, the combinations of chemicals and synthetic foods are endless.

You may be consuming appropriate amounts of water and fresh produce but absolutely love colored gum drops, sprinkles on your doughnut, and colorful ice cream, while your neighbor may only eat sandwiches from a delicatessen and drink diet soda and no water at all. Cellular damage is occurring in both of these situations and will most likely present as two different diseases.

Each Person has a Unique Chemical Cocktail

"Chemical cocktail" is a term I use to describe the unique mixture of all the different synthetic ingredients a person consumes. Prescription medications, artificial coffee creamers, fast foods, synthetic cereal bars, candies, and salty snacks are a few examples of synthetic foodstuffs. *Because the choices are so great, rarely will two people ever consume the exact same chemical cocktail.* They may be similar, but they will rarely be the same. This principal is also true for combinations of antioxidants, vitamins, and minerals. No two people will have the same levels of the "good stuff" to combat and remove the toxins that are in their bodies. With all the combinations for chemical consumption, new diseases and new forms of cancer will continue to surface and be named.

Prescription medications are a synthetic, toxic, growing addition to our culture. The United States does not have a tea culture or a natural medicine culture, we have a POP culture: POP-a-pill instead of eating correctly or soda-POP to take the place of water or POP-in-a-movie instead of taking a walk. True health is not encouraged. Destruction of health is marketed in every aspect of American life.

Natural medicine and holistic practices are still a prominent way of life in Afghanistan, Albania, Algeria, Antigua, Argentina, Armenia, Aruba, Australia, Austria, Azerbaijan, Argentina, Asia, Bahamas, Bahrain, Bangladesh, Barbados, Belgium, Belize, Bermuda, Bolivia, Bosnia, Brazil, Bulgaria, Canada, Chile, China, Colombia, Costa Rica, Cuba, Cyprus, Czech Republic, Denmark, Dominica, Dominican Republic, Eastern Europe, Ecuador, Egypt, Estonia, Ethiopia, Fiji, Finland, France, Germany, Greece, Greenland, Grenada, Guatemala, Guyana, Haiti, Honduras, Hungary, Iceland, India, Indonesia, Iran, Iraq, Ireland, Italy, Jamaica, Japan, Jordan, Latin America, Kazakhstan, Kenya, North Korea, South Korea, Kosovo, Kuwait, Laos, Latvia, Lebanon, Libya, Liechtenstein, Lithuania, Luxembourg, Malaysia, Maldives, Martinique, Mexico, Mongolia, Moldova, Monaco, Montserrat, Morocco, Nepal, Netherlands, New Zealand, Nicaragua, Nigeria, Norway, Oman, Pakistan, Panama, Paraguay, Peru, Philippines, Poland, Portugal, Puerto Rico, Qatar, Romania, Russia, Saint Lucia, Saint Vincent, Saint Maarten, San Marino, Saudi Arabia, Scotland, Serbia, Singapore, Slovakia, Slovenia, South Africa, Spain, Sri Lanka, Sudan, Suriname, Sweden, Switzerland, Syria, Taiwan, Tanzania, Trinidad, Tunisia, Turkey, Turks and Caicos Islands, Ukraine, United Arab Emirates, United Kingdom, Uruguay, Venezuela, Vietnam, and Yemen. This is not a complete list; the list is vast.

One would think that with the majority of the world using natural remedies, quite successfully I might add, that we, as a melting pot representing every nationality, would embrace a more holistic approach to health.

When people are not feeling well and cannot deduce what is wrong, they make an appointment to see their medical doctor. This is what we are socially trained to do. In most cases, they leave the medical office with a prescription for a medication that rarely corrects the issue. Instead, the prescription medication adds to the toxic overload that prompted them not to feel well before they went to the medical center.

Without reviewing the nutritional content of a person's diet, a prescription medication will only mask the real cause of the ill feeling. The side effects of the medication will produce an additional drain on the body and create more symptoms. As the person's health continues to decline, more medications will be prescribed. Disease comes from cellular destruction. The cells can only be healthy when they are receiving nutrition. Prescription medications create disease—they are toxins.

Let us discuss fibromyalgia, for example. *There is no medical test to determine the presence of fibromyalgia.* It is a condition *believed* to be overactive nerves, but is not a proven fact. The diagnosis for fibromyalgia is based on symptoms and a physician's best guess after hearing a person's account of the symptoms. The result is a life-long regimen of prescription medication. In natural medicine, fibromyalgia is not a disease at all. It is the complication of toxicity in the body. The unexplained pain is *real.* The patient, of course, is feeling the symptoms they describe. The prescription medication reduces the pain but it does not cure anything. It merely masks the problem of toxicity that the body is effectively communicating through pain and fatigue. The body is revealing that it is so overburdened with toxins that it cannot feel well.

Rather than suggesting a diet filled with antioxidants and nutrition, the patient is prescribed medication with side effects that will require another prescription medication in the future.

I watched a group of foreign tourists making fun of Americans when they visited and saw the prescription medication commercials.

After hearing commercials stating that fibromyalgia is *thought* to be overactive nerves and acid reflux is *thought* to be the result of your body creating excess stomach acid, they asked, "What happens here? An American goes to bed and develops overactive nerves? The next night they go to bed and develop excess stomach acid?" And then they laughed as they inquired, "The next night, do they grow extra fingers?" Their laughter then became unstoppable as another gentleman in their party added, "No! They grow an extra chin!"

We, as Americans, are supposed to be the most progressive nation in the world and yet we ignore the basic fundamentals of nutrition and eating for health known around the world. Americans, as a whole, are overweight and unhealthy.

Prescription medications are advertised on television in the same manner as a board game you would buy for family night or a plumbing company you would call to fix your sink. Along with the long list of side effects, you are encouraged to ask your physician if the advertised medication is right for you. There is a fine line between needing a medication and wanting one.

Americans are spoiled with convenience. The true cost for that perceived convenience is disease. Rather than eating carrots and celery for a snack, it is preferred to purchase a synthetic, non-nutritional snack from a vending machine and then take a medication for the disease it creates.

The long list of side effects is proof that the medication can cause cellular destruction. The commercials tell you that the prescription medication may weaken your ability to fight infection—and it is taken anyway! The immune function in your body is a priceless commodity. Without a strong immune system, you can fall victim to any number of sicknesses.

If you are already fighting a disease, your immune system is already weak. By neglecting the risk of side effects nearly every medication possesses, Americans receive a quick, easy, and guilt-free answer. It is as if no respect for the human body exists at all.

When health begins to fail, someone or something else is to blame. Among that list are genes inherited from a relative, stresses associated with jobs and family commitments, and rarely does anyone ever admit that they destroyed their own existence because they did not have the desire to consume an appropriate diet.

People have their own will and destroy their own existence willingly by ignoring the rules of nature and the basic requirements for optimum human longevity. Nature has provided an incredible variety of fruits, vegetables, seeds, nuts, meats and fish, and herbs and teas of all varieties that are packed with nutrients. They were provided to us for food in a non-GMO, non-synthetic, chemical-free, uncontaminated box called Earth.

Great health for the remainder of your life is waiting for you. Choose to take the first step toward better health by examining your food choices.

Synthetic Food Additives

Now that you understand how the body works and the nutrients required for a healthy existence, this section will examine the contaminants in the standard American diet (SAD). You will learn how to identify them, understand the health complications they present, and how to make better choices when it comes to food purchases. Only through education and change can you preserve your right to a healthy life.

Understanding the synthetic components of food products helps you make more informed decisions about your purchases. Many people believe that if it is for sale on the grocery shelves, it is safe to consume. While one serving of a product containing one or more synthetic ingredients will not compromise your health, the majority of shoppers are ingesting large quantities of synthetic foodstuffs every day and at every meal. This is the behavior that results in disease.

The following list highlights some of the synthetic chemical additives and preservatives that are banned in other countries or have been proven to cause ill health effects.

Food Dyes

Artificial colors and flavors are synthetic, chemically created additives in over 80 percent of pre-packaged foods, fast foods, beverages and in every variety of meat products. The most commonly used food dyes in the United States are: FD&C Blue No. 1; FD&C Blue No. 2; FD&C Red No. 3; FD&C Red No. 40; FD&C Yellow No. 5; and FD&C Yellow No. 6.

Citrus Red 2 and Orange B are used to color orange peels, hot dogs, and sausage casings. These food dyes are only allowed by the FDA for limited use. We already learned in Chapter 6 that hot dogs and sausages are listed by the World Health Organization as *a top carcinogenic agent.*

Could you have ever imagined that purchasing fresh, delicious oranges for vitamin C content to help you get through cold and flu season would result in the consumption of a limited-use food dye?

Food dyes can easily be recognized by reading the label and are the most common food additives. When parents make choices for their children at the grocery market, the cereals, fruit rolls, toaster pastries, candies, juice boxes, pre-packaged lunch box selections and the variety of other items marketed for children contain food dyes and other synthetic ingredients.

These food dyes are banned in the following countries:

- Austria - Yellow #5, Yellow #6
- Finland - Blue #1
- France - Blue #1
- Norway - Blue #1, Yellow #5, Yellow #6
- United Kingdom - Red #40 is labeled "not recommended for children"

While this list of countries banning food dyes may not appear all that impressive, please keep in mind that the eating habits in these countries do not rely on pre-packaged foods in the same manner as Americans. Considering these food dyes are dangerous enough to be banned in countries where pre-packaged foods are not purchased and used as regularly as in the United States, this limited list makes a huge statement.

Food dyes are responsible for allergies, asthma, and impaired development in children.

Brominated vegetable oil (BVO) is used in sodas and sport drinks and *is banned in more than 100 countries.* BVO can build up in the liver and kidney tissues causing health complications. If you must drink a soda, read the label. Should you find brominated vegetable oil listed as an ingredient, please consider leaving that product sitting on the shelf. Your health is worth so much more than $1.99.

Azodicarbonamide can be found in a variety of breads, bread products, and baked goods in the United States. This food additive is banned in the majority of European countries and Australia. *In Singapore, they take a much stronger stance and a different approach for banning this additive: the penalty for using it is fifteen years in prison and fines up to nearly $500,000.* Azodicarbonamide is normally used in foamed plastics production, but some fast food chains have used it in their meat.[2]

Potassium Bromate is banned in Canada, China, Europe, and a warning label is required in California for products containing this ingredient. It is used in baked goods, breads, and bread products in the United States. An article published in 1999 alerting consumers about the dangers of potassium bromate, was published by the Center for Science in the Public Interest entitled "Consumer Group Calls for Ban on 'Flour Improver' Potassium Bromate Termed a Cancer Threat." In 1999, the Food and Drug Administration heard these concerns and dismissed them because it was inconvenient at the time. It is still used in products in the United States today. If you have eaten a sandwich in a fast food restaurant recently, you probably ingested potassium bromate.

Sodium nitrites are used as a preservative and flavoring, among other uses, in processed meats and other foods. It is also used in the production of fertilizers, road salt, and solid rocket propellant. *These nitrites are so dangerous that the World Health Organization listed the foods they are most commonly used in—bacon, hot dogs, sausages, and salami* - in the same carcinogenic category as cigarettes, alcohol, asbestos, arsenic, and plutonium.

Aspartame is considered another extremely dangerous food additive. It causes damage to the neurons in the brain. It is an easily recognizable ingredient in food items and beverages labeled diet, light, low-calorie, and sugar free. You would be hard pressed to find breath mints without this ingredient. Consumption of aspartame has been associated with headaches and migraines, memory loss, heart palpitations, seizures, Alzheimer's disease, depression and anxiety, as well as other health issues. Continued consumption of this food additive can cause serious medical concerns. In addition to other dangers, consuming aspartame causes you to gain weight by disrupting the signaling system in your brain. Your body is requesting nutrients and you are replacing them with toxins that create dependence. Aspartame creates weight gain, not weight loss as many people believe.

rBGH or rBST hormones are used as bovine growth hormones and are banned in Argentina, Australia, Canada, Israel, Japan, New Zealand, and Russia and require specific cautionary labeling in the European Union. These hormones have been linked to cancer and a variety of reproductive health issues. The public concern about these hormones in milk production have prompted companies to inform their customers if they are using milk in their products or selling milk containing rBGH or rBST hormones. Because there are no labeling practices in place in the United States to identify if the product originated from bovine given these hormones, businesses have taken it upon themselves to announce if their products are free from these hormones as a matter of customer service.

High fructose corn syrup is used in just about every processed food requiring sweetener. Some commercials were created to inform the public not to worry about this substance! Often, concerns about high fructose corn syrup are dismissed by those who say, "It's made from corn, and corn is as natural as sugar." High fructose corn syrup is not recognized in the body as a healthy, natural substance and it aids in declining health, especially contributing to obesity. There is nothing natural about high fructose corn syrup. Considering 89 percent of corn in the United States is genetically modified, the health consequences are unsettling. Diabetes, arthritis, and complications of the liver and kidneys are a few of the associated health complications when consuming high fructose corn syrup.

Monosodium glutamate (MSG) has a variety of names on food labels and is used as a flavoring agent. Known as monosodium glutamate, it can also appear on the label as autolyzed yeast, autolyzed yeast extract, calcium caseinate, gelatin, glutamate, glutamate acid, hydrolyzed protein, malt extract, maltodextrin, monopotassium glutamate, natural pork or beef flavor, soy protein, protease, protein fortified, textured protein, ultra-pasteurized, and yeast extract. MSG is an addictive substance that creates an urge to consume more of the product than a person would typically consume without the presence of MSG. It is difficult to locate processed food items that do not contain MSG or a derivative or MSG. MSG can cause unlimited health conditions depending on your consumption of MSG and the combination of your chemical cocktail. MSG is usually the culprit associated with diarrhea after eating Chinese take-out, for example. It is toxic inside the body.

Carrageenan is a food additive derived from seaweed. It sounds safe because it comes from a plant but that, unfortunately, is not the case. The body does not recognize the seaweed extract as a whole plant substance, rather, the chemical structure of the carrageenan extract becomes a toxin inside the body. Carrageenan is found in non-dairy products, nearly all non-organic coffee creamers, yogurts, and baked goods using non-dairy products in lieu of milk. The negative health effects associated with consuming carrageenan are chronic inflammation of every part of the body including the heart, blood vessels, nerves, joints and kidneys, irritation of the stomach and intestinal tract, and weakened immune system.

Butylated Hydroxyanisole (BHA) and Butylated Hydroxytoluene (BHT) are used as preservatives in cereals and packaged goods. They are banned in some European countries and pregnant and lactating women are encouraged to limit or completely avoid consumption of products containing BHA and BHT. These additives are listed as a possible carcinogen in California.

The listed food additives banned in other countries are just an introduction to the dangers lurking in your foods. These additives interfere with every function in the body and are the number one reason the obesity rates are climbing in the United States. Food additives complicate digestion and confuse the brain. The body does not know what to do with these foreign substances, so they get stored as fat.

Chemically manufactured food additives and preservatives exist in every food group in the grocery market unless it is a USDA certified organic product. More than 3,000 different chemicals are added to food in the United States.

You cannot possess good health and eat pre-packaged foods. Avoiding synthetic and chemically manufactured foods will help minimize your chances of experiencing weight gain, Alzheimer's disease, cancer, diabetes and heart disease, kidney disease, Crohn's disease, constipation, acne, depression, anxiety, arthritis, respiratory infections, fibromyalgia symptoms, headaches and migraines, and a variety of other health afflictions. If it is not found in nature, you are ingesting a substance that will, over time, adversely affect your health.

You will not suffer enormous health repercussions if you eat a bowl of non-organic ice cream twice a year. It is when you review your grocery purchases, however, that you may realize that nearly every item you are ingesting poses an immediate threat to your health. Furthermore, when your health begins to fail because of synthetic consumption, the medical community will view your symptoms as disease and prescribe a synthetic medication to address the symptoms instead of removing the cause.

9

Changing Your Eating Habits—Step-by-Step Process

Changing any habit is difficult—but changing how you eat, when you eat it, and what you eat is a major undertaking! I was visiting a friend in the hospital after she was in a car accident. She was in a semi-private room, which was not very private. I overheard the conversation from the patient in the other bed as she was talking to her father. She was just diagnosed with cancer after X-rays were taken immediately following a near-fatal vehicle accident. As the conversation went on, I concluded that the father was a United States Marine.

His comments were incredible. He told her she could beat cancer by juicing and taking high doses of vitamin C because he witnessed it in Colorado. Her response was asking how long she had to do that because she didn't like vegetables. His reply granted her permission to explore natural health options. He told her that he watched her become a star basketball player even though she was not the tallest one on the team. He watched her excel in every subject while she was in school and away at college. He told her he would be by her side every step of the way as he helped her fight cancer without chemotherapy. He promised that he would be able to watch her fulfill every dream she ever had because, more than anyone else he had ever met, she had more strength, determination, and conviction to accomplish anything she set her mind to do. He told her he knew she could beat her cancer diagnosis and even though she did not wear the uniform, she was one of the few.

She cried out loud. Tears rolled down my face on the other side of the curtain. His response to her cancer diagnosis was to never give up. He encouraged her without placing any blame and offered her a way to deal with a scary, life-threatening situation. The words he constructed came from his heart and helped her to believe she could defeat cancer.

I do not know what happened to this young lady. I do know that her support system was unshakable.

Changing your life takes determination. When I am weary or complacent about any goal in my life, I remember this man's words. Not only did he encourage his daughter, he encouraged my friend to overcome her injuries and encouraged me to press on regardless of trying circumstances.

I hope this story encourages you, too. I hope he buys this book and reaches out to me! My words may not be as profound as the Marine's, but hopefully by providing a manageable step-by-step process, you will be able to adjust to these necessary life changes without feeling confused or miserable. Please know that every positive change you make is a giant step toward better health.

Step 1 - Change your milk purchase to USDA certified organic 1 percent milk.

When you go to the grocery market to make this purchase, look at the expiration date on non-organic milk. The expiration is dated out approximately ten to fourteen days. When you look at the organic milk, it will be dated out four to six weeks! The *chemicals* in non-organic milk are what make it go rancid, not the milk itself. Certified Organic milk does not contain chemicals, synthetics, hormones or steroids, therefore, does not expire in ten to fourteen days.

Not only will you notice that the certified organic milk tastes better, you will not experience stomach issues that many people associate with being lactose intolerant. The vast majority of people who think they are lactose intolerant are reacting to the unlisted chemical by-products of non-organic milk.

Replacing the milk you currently purchase with organic milk is an easy place to start and provides immediate relief for many people who consume milk daily. I believe that the hormones and other chemicals given to cows adversely affect fertility and sexual performance in both men and women in the United States because they are still present in the milk.

Consuming 1 percent organic milk offers nutritional benefits without the additional calories and fat. Use organic milk instead of coffee creamer to eliminate additional chemicals in your diet.

Step 2 – Eat raw, certified organic fruit for breakfast.

Fruit is full of nutrients and natural juices that will fully digest in one to two hours. The nutrients will fortify every cell in your body.

There is such a variety of fresh organic fruits that you can choose the ones you prefer. Choose different fruits each week to vary your nutritional intake.

The price tag scares people at first. Certified organic apples are smaller than genetically modified apples and the price is higher. An entire bag of certified organic apples may cost $4.99 - $5.99 but are packed with nutrients and contains no synthetic components. Most people spend more than the price of a bag of organic apples on a breakfast sandwich and a coffee each morning, which provides no nutritional value at all. Remember that it is not how much you eat that satisfies hunger, it is the nutrient content of what you eat.

Step 3 – Eliminate all brightly colored artificial snacks from your home and office.

This step will remove temptation and remove alternatives for that organic fresh fruit you just purchased that can double as a sweet, delicious snack.

These products are toxic to your body. They do not contain nutrition and will disrupt the proper digestion of the nutritious food you have eaten. They contribute to diabetes and other illnesses, cost money that can be spent on highly nutritious food choices, and by eliminating your favorite junk-food snacks, you take a huge leap toward committing yourself to better health. Step 3 is more difficult for most people than Steps 1 and 2.

Step 4 – Eliminate all soda (carbonated soft drinks).

Sodas promote tooth decay, diabetes, kidney disease, and inhibit liver and immune function. They are a costly expenditure with zero benefit to your well-being.

Step 5 – Replace all cabinet foods and refrigerated condiments with organic choices, if necessary.

Nearly half of everyone choosing to follow this protocol expressed that their stash of refrigerated condiments were past the expiration date so they would have to throw them in the garbage any way! When eating fresh fruits and vegetables, many cabinet foods and condiments are an unnecessary purchase. If they have been there for a while, you were not using them to start with. Replacing them is not necessary and you gain the space they occupied and can use it to store other items like organic tea and organic spices.

Once your body adjusts to nutrient-packed fruits and vegetables, your desire for packaged foods diminishes greatly. When you eliminate synthetic extras from your diet, you will save money, calories, and eliminate ingesting harmful toxins.

As you consume nutritious choices, you will lose weight, feel less hungry, and gravitate toward an overall healthier lifestyle. It takes a very limited amount of time to serve organic fruits, salads, home-made raw soups, or grilled fish and steamed vegetables for dinner than eating out or making a conventional, standard American meal. Making this change will leave adequate time for much needed exercise, even if it is only a brief ten-minute walk, time for relaxation, and time for sleep. As an added bonus, there are also fewer dishes, pots, and pans to scrub after dinner.

Change is not easy and is the only reason people continually live a miserable lifestyle. The idea of forsaking their daily routine is uncertain and scary. For others, it is a condition of merely making up their minds that there is a better way to live and then making the changes that are necessary to change.

"Our way of thinking, our approach to health and disease, our willingness to take responsibility for our circumstances makes us—as hygienists—different. And the more consistent and persistent we are in our way of life the further from the average American we get. But there is a world of difference between normal and healthy. Normal people are sick several times a year tired most of the time, and very frequently complain of numerous ongoing ailments. They usually have aches and pains and one or more degenerative syndromes. Being normal just doesn't seem like that much fun. Decide to be different! Seek high-level health including a willingness to face whatever challenges being different presents!"

–Dr. Douglas Graham, 1986

10

Undernourished

An article in *USA Today* published on January 22, 1986, stated, "We are the most overfed yet undernourished country in the history of the world. The average person in the United States consumes 3,393 calories per day, which is phenomenal. It's the highest in the world."

When you add to this dilemma that nearly 80 percent of all packaged foods in the United States contain harmful chemicals, it is easy to realize why Americans are also the most diseased nation in the world.

The increase in cancer rates, diabetes, high blood pressure, nerve disorders, depression, birth defects, autism, learning disabilities, eczema, arthritis, sleep disorders, depression, Alzheimer's disease, Crohn's disease, Parkinson's disease, obesity, and kidney disorders have dramatically increased over the past thirty years.

Finding a household where meals are prepared with whole, natural foods are few and far between. It has become a form of entertainment to go out to eat. Because of this societal change, no one weighs the consequences of what is in the food, the negative impact the synthetic components will have, or the health disasters awaiting them in the future due to the consistent consumption of foodstuffs with no nutritional value.

Being healthy and raising healthy children begins with you. If you are preparing meals of boxed macaroni and cheese, baking frozen french fries at 450 degrees, dining at fast food restaurants, eating synthetically made breakfast cereals with non-organic milk, and feeding children synthetic snacks, you can anticipate childhood illness. These food items affect the immune system, disorient their hormones, and disrupt the healthy growth of their brain and its function. A child under the age of two does not even have the enzymes required to break down grains found in crackers, cookies, or cereals!

Investing the time and energy to read the labels and understand what chemicals you and your family are ingesting provides a foundation for good health for the rest of your lives.

School lunches are not food; they are trash. They contain little to no nutriment, are laced with chemical additives, and impair every function in the body. Yet parents kiss and hug their children and send them off to school to ingest approved chemical substances and wonder why they do not behave properly or sit still in class, cannot sleep at night, and lack motivation.

You are responsible for their health, as well as your own, with every bite. For the amount of money spent on a fast food meal, it costs less to eat certified organic products. When the body receives actual nutrition, it is not as hungry. When you feed children food with little or no nutrients, they become hungry all the time. It is not because they are pigs, it is because their bodies are asking for the nutrients required to operate and function properly. Eating anything or everything does not accomplish this requirement. Eating an apple for a snack provides nutrition, while eating a bag of potato chips does not. The body is still hungry because it is asking for nutrients, not just a food substance.

The medical community would have you believe that the majority of your health issues are inherited, but they are wrong. The majority of your health issues derive from inherited eating habits, not inherited genes.

In the following example, challenge your knowledge of eating habits and the resulting health conditions. When I tell this story in seminars, nearly everyone can determine the outcome.

Fred is one of the nicest people you will ever meet. In his lifetime, he helped raise enough money for the local fire department to purchase four brand-new fire engines. He worked a construction job and never married. He was one of seven children and grew up on a farm. Fred's dad suffered heart disease and his mother had life-threatening diabetes. Fred had a standard routine every week. He would eat eggs, home fries, bacon, and white toast with jelly at the local diner every day. He washed it down with four to five cups of black coffee. He would leave the diner, go down the street, buy a pack of cigarettes and two 20-ounce bottles of soda and drive to work.

Lunch time was a hoagie made with deli ham, salami, cheese, and mayonnaise. Fred enjoyed this delicacy every working day. But dinner time was a little different each day. He either went for pizza, a chain restaurant buffet, or stopped at a fast food drive through. He did not drink water; the only beverages he drank were coffee and soda. The only fruit he consumed was a few bites of his mother's apple pie. Vegetables such as green beans, carrots, or corn he would eat along with a heaping side of potatoes, either mashed, fried, scalloped, or occasionally baked, which would require gravy.

What do you think caused Fred's demise at age 49? Did you guess heart attack or diabetes, cancer, or lung disease? Fred died of a massive heart attack while walking to his vehicle to go to the diner one morning. His daily food and drink consumption provided little to no nutritional value and contained many synthetic materials, chemicals, and other toxins; no nutrition and no water. Do you think his heart failure was an inherited gene or constant bad food choices?

When a person we love and adore passes at a young age, we look for someone or something to blame. Fred chose every day to make horrible choices when it came to food. Do you think he knew a better way to live? Fred's poor eating habits did not diminish his kindness or his loving, out-going personality. Nor did it ease the pain of his passing. It is so unfortunate that Fred was seemingly unaware that he was silently digging himself an early grave just like so many others do in this world.

"I believe the biggest mistake in United States history is the willful contamination of our food supply and the willingness of the American people to ignore it."
–DK Guyer, PhD

When we review the amount of chemical exposure we experience on a daily basis, it becomes overwhelming. Here is a look at the chemical exposure you may experience throughout a normal day. You get out of bed and it begins:

Toothpaste
Deodorant
Mouthwash
Shampoo
Conditioner
Soap or shower gel
Hand soap
Hairspray
Shaving cream
Cologne
Lotion
Nail polish
Nail polish remover
Make up
Make up remover
Acne products
Dental floss
Contact lens solution
Medication
You dress in your clothes washed in chemicals.
Eat breakfast on dishes washed with chemicals.
Your breakfast foods *are* chemicals.
Your coffee has chemicals.
Your coffee creamer *is* chemicals.
And you haven't made it out of the house yet!

Then you eat non-organic, chemical-laced foodstuffs all day long, drink soda, and take home carry-out food or order something for delivery. When you are consuming synthetic foods all day long on a daily basis, good health cannot be achieved or maintained.

According to a report from the United States Department of Agriculture Economic Research Service dated November 2016, 89 percent of corn, 89 percent of cotton, and 94 percent of soybeans grown in the United States are genetically modified varieties.[1]

The results of these staggering statistics for our future health are still unknown. Some form of GMO corn or soy is in nearly every processed food product. Even if you choose not to eat corn, it is used in many kinds of products. Here is a short list of products made using GMO corn:[2]

Acetic and amino acids
Antibiotics
Alcoholic beverages and brewing
Aspirin
Baby food
Bacon
Baked goods
Bakery products
Baking powder
Batteries
Blankets and bedding
Bookbinding
Breadings, coatings, batters
Candies
Cake, cookie, dessert mixes
Caramel color
Canned fruits, fruit fillings
Cardboard
Carbonated and fruit beverages
Carpet tile
Cereals
Chalk
Charcoal briquettes
Cheese spreads
Chewing gum
Citric acid
Cleaners, detergents
Coffee whitener
Coatings on paper, wood and metal
Condiments
Color carrier for printing
Corn bread
Confections, chocolate
Corn chips
Corn flakes
Cornmeal mixes
Cosmetics
Crayons
Disposable diapers
Doughnuts
Drink cups, plates and cutlery
Dried soups
Dusting for pizzas
Dyes and inks
Electroplating and galvanizing
English muffins
Fermentation processes
Enzymes
Fireworks
Food acids
Food coloring
Food packaging
Fritters
Frosting and icing
Frozen and dried eggs
Frozen pudding
Glues and adhesives
Gravy mixes
Hams
Hot dogs, bologna

Ice cream and sherbets
Industrial filters and water
Industrial sweetener
Instant breakfast foods
Jams, jellies, preserves
Laminated building materials
Lubricants
Marshmallows
Meat products
Muffins
Organic solvents
Pancake mixes
Peanut butter
Pharmaceuticals
Plastics
Powdered mixes
Precooked frozen foods
Rubber tires
Salt
Seasoning mixes
Shaving cream
Snack foods
Soups
Spoon bread
Spray cooking oil
Textiles
Tomato sauces
Wallboard and wallpaper
Worcestershire sauce

Hush puppies
Industrial chemicals
Insecticides
Instant pudding mix
Instant tea
Leather tanning
Mannitol
Matches
Metal plating
Ore and oil refining
Paints
Paper, recycled paper
Pet food
Pickles and relishes
Potato chips
Powdered sugar
Rayon
Salad dressings
Sausage
Shampoo
Shoe polish
Soaps and cleaners
Spice mixes
Sports & active wear
Surgical dressings
Theatrical makeup
Vinegar
Wine
Yeast

What a list. All of these products contain genetically modified corn. We use them. We consume some of them. We think nothing of it.

There was a saying about how well the corn was progressing in the field when I was growing up: "It should be knee high by the Fourth of July." The corn was supposed to be knee high, about two feet, by Independence Day. Most of the time, the weeds were taller than the corn by then! Today, corn is seven to eight feet tall by July Fourth and the weeds do not exist in the corn field anymore. Thanks to Genetically Modified Organisms (GMO), the corn is "Roundup® ready" when it is planted. That means that the corn DNA has been genetically modified to resist the herbicide Roundup, the corn will still grow in the fields treated with Roundup, and when humans consume the modified corn, traces of Roundup can be found inside the body. If you regularly consume corn products, the traces of Roundup can accumulate in your body based on heavy consumption of corn. The severe health consequences of consuming GMO corn and corn products will not be known and confirmed for some time. What we do know is the human body was designed to eliminate or fight toxic substances.

FDA Approval of Chemical Compounds

Today we see the results of contamination and lack of research prior to federal approval for medications through the following types of television commercials. A variety of legal groups representing people negatively affected by harmful chemicals and medications state, "If you or a loved one has suffered serious side effects or even death from the prescription drug named ____________, contact the toll free number at the bottom of your screen." These types of commercials are continually advising us that an approved medical product or prescription drug has caused irreversible health damage and that a lawsuit is pending.

The following is a list of some of the FDA approved prescription drugs that were later removed from the market due to their dangerous health effects.

Prempro - hormone replacement
Ortho Evra - birth control patch
Seroquel - anti-psychotic
Neurontin - anti-seizure
Yasmin - birth control
Avandia - diabetes
Vioxx - pain killer

OrLAAM - opioid dependence
Raplon - neuromuscular blocker in anesthesia
Baycol - cholesterol
Mylotarg - acute myeloid leukemia
Seldane - allergies
Xigris - sepsis
Meridia - obesity
Palladone - pain killer
Darvon/Darvocet - pain killer
Zelnorm - IBS/constipation
NeurtroSpec - imaging aid for diagnosing appendicitis
Raptiva - psoriasis
Permax - Parkinson's disease

The purpose of listing some of the withdrawn prescription medications is to illustrate that not everything available on the market using chemicals and synthetically made substances is safe, even if it has been FDA approved. The common misconception is that medication, even when the side effects are verbally listed on television commercials, is still safe and that the side effects will not happen to you.

The same misconception applies to synthetic and chemical ingredients in the food supply. Many of the synthetic and chemical ingredients that have been approved by the FDA were based on the assumption that the product would be consumed in single serving sizes only. For example: one 12-ounce can of diet soda is a serving, not a 2-liter bottle; twelve to sixteen chips is the serving size for tortilla chips, not half of the bag; a half cup is a serving size for ice cream, not a quart! While the FDA approved these chemicals compounds, it was never intended for daily consumption or the total replacement of fresh fruits, vegetables, and water.

To demonstrate that the intended product was legitimately safe using the guidelines for FDA approval, let's look at diet soda again. One 12-ounce serving of diet soda while consuming an appropriate diet is considered safe. Consuming half of a 2-liter bottle of diet soda was not part of the consideration for FDA approval, and therefore, the overconsumption of this product cannot reflect poorly on the FDA's approval of the product. When an individual decides to consume diet soda in excess and/or in place of water, and becomes ill, the FDA does not accept responsibility for that individual's negligent actions.

The FDA does not have the responsibility to recall or reconsider its approval of this substance because the consumer is using it irresponsibly. The serving size for any product is clearly listed on the label.

An FDA approval of a substance is interpreted by the American population as an undisputed seal of safety. Because of the safety approval, Americans believe they can consume all they want of a synthetic product without negative health consequences. They are then surprised to learn that synthetic products cause disease. New and rare forms of cancer and disease are being uncovered at a rapid rate. They are all the result of synthetic eating and drinking habits, medications, overexposure to chemicals, and lack of nutrition.

There is no one item on the grocery shelves that will be responsible for your demise. One can of diet soda a year will not cause you great harm but consuming a 2-liter bottle of it in one day and eating foodstuffs with no nutrition daily will complicate your health. It is the combination of all the synthetic products being used and consumed that cause the issue. Americans are toxic waste dumps awaiting deplorable health issues.

Everyone knows that drinking a fifth of bourbon every day will cause liver damage and early death. If this is what you are doing with your life, you may be an alcoholic and will suffer the debilitating effects of alcoholism. The same is true for soda and other synthetics foods. If the only beverage you consume is soda, people around you know why you are sick. Soda, with sugar or without sugar, is not a replacement for water. Your habits are not much different from that of the person drinking the bourbon, and the alcohol that causes alcoholism is just like the sugar or caffeine that causes soda addiction. The soda habit is an addiction.

When prescription drugs were released and deemed safe for use, no one could foresee the long-term effects the new prescription drugs would have on the recipient. The same is true of the consistent chain of new chemicals being added to our food supply. You cannot predict what the outcome will be, but you do know that the human body is not designed to withstand chemicals and other toxins without disastrous side effects. You can make a difference in your health, your family's health, the health of a friend or coworker, and even the health of future generations by changing what you buy, what you eat, and how you approach the use of chemicals and synthetics in your daily routine.

"I believe that if we refuse to make serious changes and serious choices when it comes to our eating habits and our lifestyle choices, our grandchildren will be born with irreversible health effects."

–DK Guyer, PhD

11

Acid Reflux

Antacid sales surpass $2 billion a year in the United States, supporting an undeniable statement about our health, our horrific eating habits, and our state of mind. In this section, I will demonstrate how easily acid reflux, heartburn, and indigestion can be extinguished—for most people—for the remainder of your life without purchasing any antacid products. You will gain understanding of what causes this type of discomfort, why the body reacts to certain foods, and why it is paramount that you change some of your eating habits now to avoid more serious consequences in the future.

The standard American diet (SAD) is an oversized culinary disaster! Quarter-pound hamburgers with bacon, cheese, mayonnaise, tomato, lettuce, ketchup, and mustard are not nutritional choices. Many of these monster sandwiches contain 850 to 950 calories, 50-60 g fat, 200-250 g cholesterol and 1,800-2,000 mg sodium. The worst part about the standard American meal is that four out of five people inhale their food without properly chewing it up before swallowing it. French fries are devoured by the hands full, not one at a time. Soda is chugged down and the cup is refilled at least once, if not multiple times.

Some people believe that at some point in their lives, their bodies will all of the sudden begin to develop excess stomach acid. This is an untruth that many people blame for their acid reflux issues.

This is what truly happens inside the body when acid reflux occurs. Let's imagine that your stomach is the size of a 16-ounce, see-through plastic water bottle. Approximately one third to one half of the bottle filled with water would represent the average amount of stomach acid. Now imagine adding a quarter pound hamburger with all the extras and a large order of french fries being semi-chewed and stuffed into the bottle. Then add a 20-ounce soda on top of that. At what point will the water bottle begin to overflow? When the overflow point is reached, the stomach acid has been pushed to the upper limits of the stomach into the esophagus.

Now if you make a fist, this is a more accurate representation of the size of the stomach. Most people eat four to five times more food at one sitting than can fit into their stomach and it is rarely ever properly chewed before being swallowed. The stomach acid becomes very active trying to break down the huge amount of partially chewed food in the stomach. Then heartburn and indigestion occur.

Now, let's imagine the quarter-pound hamburger, french fries, and soda was the lunchtime meal. It will take approximately ten to twelve hours to digest the improperly masticated food stuffs. Before the first meal has been fully digested from lunch, the next meal is being consumed at dinner. Steak, mashed potatoes, gravy, a roll or piece of bread, canned green beans smothered in margarine, and a delicious piece of cherry pie, and some soda or beer. The stomach is now so stretched, and so full, the stomach acid is still very active trying to digest and break down the huge amount of half-chewed food. Feeling the discomfort of eating too much, the average American takes an antacid. Within an hour or two, more food will be consumed. Ice cream, popcorn, candy, beer, soda, chips, cookies, and a variety of other snacks items are forced into the already compromised digestive system. The stomach acid increases to accommodate the excessive amount of hard-to-digest foodstuffs waiting to be digested.

Overeating creates one problem. Food that has barely been chewed at all before it is swallowed is another problem. Combining all the food groups together in one meal creates another issue. Few people are aware that digestive enzymes perform different functions and at different times. The digestive enzyme, pepsin, works to break down protein in the stomach. When protein is present, pepsin, a highly acidic digestive enzyme, breaks down proteins into various amino acids.

Protein digestion takes precedence over carbohydrate digestion. Carbohydrates cannot be digested until the pepsin has subsided in the stomach. To better explain the acids and their purpose, let's think about it this way: If you eat eggs, hash browns, and toast for breakfast, a chicken sandwich for lunch, and a burrito with a side of chips and queso for dinner, how would the digestive enzymes handle the digestion process for all of this food?

Protein always gets precedence in the digestive process. The hydrochloric acid present in the stomach is a relatively neutral acid and helps facilitate the action of pepsin. The eggs for breakfast are just completing their digestion when the chicken arrives. The stomach has not yet completed digesting the chicken when the beef arrives from the burrito. Since pepsin is highly acidic, the nearly neutral hydrochloric acid used for digesting the starches, cannot complete its job. The toast and potatoes from this morning's meal have not yet been properly digested. Neither is the roll from lunch. They begin to decompose or ferment in the stomach rather than being fully digested because the stomach is consistently being filled with under-masticated proteins that take eight to ten hours minimum to digest.

Food Combining

The process of eating properly for easy digestion is called *food combining.* Simply put, proteins are consumed with non-starch vegetables. Carbohydrates are consumed with vegetables. Fruits are eaten alone. The design of our digestive process does not allow for easy digestion of foods the way Americans consume them. Many cultures eat raw, fresh fruit for breakfast. It fully digests within two hours. For lunch, vegetables are consumed with rice or pasta. The evening meal is traditionally the one containing proteins. Fresh vegetables are served with fish, chicken, veal, or beef. When utilizing the food combining rules, digestion becomes easy and the body benefits from the efficient conversion of food to nutrition.

The average American overeats at every meal. They overeat food that contains little to no nutritional value. In actuality, their bodies are craving nutrition but receiving pounds upon pounds of useless, synthetic matter. This is the major factor that makes the United States the sickest, most diseased nation in the world.

The physician has a tough job. When you arrive at a physician's office complaining about your terrible heartburn and extreme discomfort, you are expecting a medical reason for why you are feeling so badly. The number one cause of heartburn is overeating. You are expecting a medical reason and a pill to cure your pain. The physician should tell you to cut your portion sizes in half and skip all snacks between meals, but that will not go over well. Explaining that you are consuming more food than your digestion system can handle will not be acceptable either.

Having the physician hand you a prescription to cover up the symptoms is what most people expect for daily heartburn and acid reflux conditions. The average person does not want to change their habits or be told that their eating habits are the sole reason for their misery.

Stuffing your stomach with a breakfast burrito that contains 710 calories, 47 g fat, 1,260 mg sodium, 51 g carbohydrates and an overwhelming variety of chemicals creates sluggishness, lack of concentration, and acid reflux. What is all of that doing inside your body? It is developing disease. The acid reflux pain you are experiencing is your body's way of alerting you that it is being over stuffed and compromised.

Let's look at doughnuts. They are considered a breakfast food, but are comprised of bleached flour, oils, chemicals, synthetic flavors, and are high in saturated fats. They sit like a lead sinker in your stomach. Then, on top of your favorite synthetic breakfast choice, you add 20 ounces of your favorite coffee with a totally artificial non-dairy creamer. This adds another round of synthetic junk to start the day. Yet people choose to take a pill and ignore the body's natural reaction to the constant, ridiculous over-stuffing of our incredible human body.

Acid reflux is your trophy for eating unreasonable so-called food items for your meals. Carry your antacids with pride. You earned every minute of the discomfort known as heartburn and indigestion. As harsh as this may sound, you know that it is true! You know what foods make you feel miserable and you still eat them and pay money for them and for your antacid.

Changing your habits and feeling better means you have to relinquish your well-earned acid reflux prescription for healthier choices.

Occasionally, acid reflux symptoms can occur in individuals who eat very little. The stomach shrinks and the acid erupts as the body hungers for nutrition and irritates the esophagus. Small meals throughout the day help eliminate this issue entirely.

The second most common reason for acid reflux is swallowing food before it is properly chewed. *Americans are notorious for eating too fast and not chewing their food.* This habit adds an additional strain on the digestive system. Digestion begins in the mouth when food is coated with saliva containing enzymes that prepare the food for the digestive process when it reaches the stomach. The stomach must overwork to break down the large pieces of food into small particles that can then be assimilated into nutrition in the colon. Many people experience sluggishness and lack of motivation after eating too quickly. The body is utilizing all necessary nerve energy to digest the food.

One of the most common food substances involved in acid reflux is tomato-based sauces such as barbeque sauce, pizza sauce, spaghetti sauce, salsa, hot sauce, and taco sauce. There are two major reasons for the discomfort. One, the tomatoes used in non-organic sauce are peeled with chemicals. There are only a few processors using steam in order to peel tomatoes, but the majority of tomatoes are chemically peeled. When you eat spaghetti and indigestion and heartburn ensue, stop eating it! Your body is telling you the substance is irritating to your digestive track. The second reason for the discomfort is that most dishes using tomato sauce are improperly food combined. Pizza is a combination of carbohydrates (crust), fruit (tomato sauce), cheese (protein/dairy), meat or meat substitutes (protein), and cooking oils (fat). This combination is difficult to digest even if all the ingredients were the highest quality on earth—organic.

With this wicked combination of all food groups, many people inhale three or four slices, swallow it partially chewed, and rinse it down with an ice-cold beer or soda. When the acid reflux occurs, the person decides that it is time to make another doctor appointment to increase the dose of their acid reflux prescription because it no longer works. The realization that you are a human being with nutritional requirements and not a trash bin that can house endless amounts of synthetic culinary disasters is the beginning of understanding better health and eliminating the symptoms of acid reflux forever.

"Who is strong? He that can conquer bad habits!"
–Ben Franklin, 1770

12

Attention Deficient Hyperactivity Disorder

I began tutoring other students struggling with certain subjects while I was in the eighth grade. I continued doing so until I was a junior in high school. I noticed a common denominator among the students I was tutoring: many of them were breathing through their mouths instead of through their noses. These students were not rude or belligerent as the standard stereotype today conveys of a child with Attention Deficient Hyperactivity Disorder (ADHD). They were better at sports or music, but sitting still for endless hours trying to comprehend subjects no one was really interested in learning to begin with, was even more difficult for them.

The reason for the anxious, cannot-sit-still, very distracted behavior associated with ADHD is simple. When children cannot breathe properly, their body is not getting enough oxygen. Hence, the "fight or flight" mechanism engages. When they move around a little bit, they breathe a little better. This is the built-in response that helps keep humans alive. To determine if a child truly has ADHD, have the child place a hand over his or her mouth. Ask the child to breathe through the nose for a full one minute. If the child cannot breathe through the nose or if it is too hard to get a breath that way, have the child remove his or her hand from their mouth and breathe normally. You can do this first so the child will feel comfortable with the exercise.

Please do not become alarmed if the child cannot breathe through the nose. Be overjoyed! You now have the ability to change the child's health for the better for the remainder of life.

The two conditions that inhibit proper breathing are a deviated septum or enlarged tonsils and adenoids. While I am not an advocate for surgery, these surgeries are minimally invasive and correct a physical condition that will eliminate a lifetime of prescription medications and many resulting side effects. As soon as the child recovers from the surgery, his or her attention span will increase, the child will be able to sleep through the night, and will have better health because the child's body is getting appropriate oxygen.

**The information about the correlation between ADHD symptoms and inhibited breathing has not been scientifically proven. This is my sole observation after witnessing countless children and adults with breathing issues and receiving an ADHD diagnosis.*

When children can breathe through their noses properly and they are exhibiting signs of ADHD, check their diet. Nine out of ten children are nutritionally deficient—especially in magnesium — and are experiencing the side effects of artificial food dyes and synthetic foods. Eliminate synthetic foods and sugar and watch them as they regain focus and a good night's sleep with proper nutrition, water, and sufficient rest.

While a medically diagnosed ADHD child may seem distracting and unmanageable by a teacher, please keep in mind that children were never designed to be inside a schoolroom for seven hours a day sitting still, humankind decided it should be that way. Just because children are distracted does not mean there is something wrong with them.

Children are each born with their own gifts. Each child excels in different subjects. We are all designed that way and each of us has our strengths. In a classroom, however, each child is expected to contribute, excel, and respond in the same general fashion.

Stresses at home causing worry and lack of sleep are a very real contributing factor for attention deficit. When a child's grandparent is dying of cancer or marital issues are disrupting family life, the child may not be capable of paying attention. This situation does not require ADHD medication. It requires compassion.

School lunches are low-cost, synthetic, non-nutritional, artificial excuses for food. Hot dogs, bacon, and sausage are listed by the World Health Organization as known carcinogens in humans. These items, as well as other substances banned around the world, have no place being served to our students as food. Parents and teachers should be working together to eliminate hazardous environments for children that includes their food consumption. It takes a village to raise a child and children are the result of that village. Start the awareness and pack a healthy lunch for your child and encourage other parents to do the same.

Adult ADHD has the same components. Many adults taking prescription medications for the symptoms of ADHD are also using Continuous Positive Airway Pressure (CPAP) machines to help them breath while sleeping. This machine "forces air into the nasal passages at pressures high enough to overcome obstructions in the airway and stimulate normal breathing."[1]

The majority of attention deficit disorders can be remedied by consuming a diet free from artificial flavors, artificial colorings, fast food and sugar, analyzing unusual circumstances contributing to attention deficit and acquiring appropriate amounts of oxygen. To me, the correlation is very evident—lack of focus equals lack of oxygen and proper nutrition.

13

Cancer

The word "cancer" strikes a fear in people unlike any other word. To many, it means they have to fight a battle against a raging enemy they cannot see, with an army of people they have never met, leading them into unknown territory without any knowledge, training, or weapons. The thought of cancer living and breeding inside your body is not a pleasant one.

Heart disease is the number one killer in the United States. Cancer is the second. Nearly 30 percent of all cancer deaths could have been prevented by eliminating cigarette smoking, excessive alcohol intake, refined sugar intake, obesity, a diet of little to no nutrition, inactivity, and appropriate education about health and nutrition prior to stage four cancer diagnoses. The remaining 60 percent of cancers are coupled with other life-threatening diseases such as heart, liver, kidney, and blood disease. Since heart disease is the most predominant health issue, I will use it as an example.

Persons with heart disease are medicated with synthetic compounds to extend their life. Rather than utilizing a diet to restore health, these persons continue to eat whatever they want any time of the day and night and complicate their heart issues to the limits of prescription medication. The combination of the consistent chemical ingestion leads to cancer. The heart issue is now so elevated that removing prescription medication from the equation is no longer a viable option. These persons need to remain on their prescription medication until either their heart fails or the cancer envelopes their life. While the World Health

Organization estimates 30 percent of cancers can be eliminated by following their suggestions, I estimate that it is closer to 60 percent if heart disease, diabetes, and kidney disease can be reversed at the early stages through diet instead of prescription medications.

Let's examine how cancer evolves inside the body. A beautiful, bright-eyed baby girl named Sophie, is born in the city. Both her parents have professional jobs. Her father is a lawyer and her mother is a marketing executive. Her mother returns to work six weeks after Sophie is born. Sophie is taken to child care where she is fed infant formula (synthetics), and at six months old, she is given several vaccinations (synthetics). Sophie also begins eating baby foods (pureéd preservatives and synthetics). By the time Sophie is one year old, she has already breathed diesel fumes, gas fumes, pollutants, and second-hand smoke during her stroller rides on the sidewalks down the heavily traveled city streets.

At two years old, Sophie is hugging the dog treated with chemicals, walking, crawling, playing and eating on the floor cleaned with chemicals, bathed in and fed with chemicals, and is well on her way to developing a sugar habit. Another year passes and she is now old enough to eat an array of soft foods in a restaurant. Sophie's parents enjoy taking their bundle of joy out with them on the weekends because they spend limited time with her during the week.

When her professional parents hear that Sophie has cancer shortly after her eighth birthday, they are mortified. Sophie's school lunches were pre-packaged, her dinners were Chinese takeout, pizza, burgers and fries, soda, hoagies, drive-thru kids meals, artificially-colored and flavored juice boxes, ice cream, and candy. Sophie's tiny body was riddled with too many toxins and not enough nutrition. Of course, Sophie's parents would take her to the highest rated doctors for her chemotherapy because their daughter, Sophie, deserved the best.

It tears me up inside to watch loving parents hand over their diet soda for their toddler to drink. Children in the United States are fed boxed macaroni and cheese, colorful cereals, juice boxes, french fries, pizza, and cheeseburgers as soon as they have enough teeth to eat them. Social media is plastered with requests to pray for sick children. Every life is precious. Every single life is a gift. Children do not possess the knowledge to make better choices about the foods they consume. Providing children with synthetic, brightly colored sugars is a proven path to the destruction of their health.

Cancer is cancer. It does not discriminate against age, race, ethnicity, religion, marital status, gender, sexual orientation, hair color, nationality, economic status, or political affiliation. Cancer is cancer. The more toxins you ingest, the faster the cancer diagnosis arrives.

If you are already diagnosed with heart disease and high cholesterol and are taking medications for these health complications, you seriously need to consider a diet change immediately. The heart disease is telling you the body is having serious side effects because you are eating high-cholesterol, high-sodium, low-nutrition meals. The cancer-come-and-get-me stage is already set.

Eating five or more fast food or takeout meals in a week sets the stage for cancer because those five meals in the United States provide more chemicals and synthetic toxins than your body can process and remove before cells begin to deteriorate. Twenty fast food or restaurant meals in a month equates to disastrous health complications. Rather than changing their eating habits, most people opt to address the symptoms of heartburn or acid reflux, insomnia, constipation, hypertension, diabetes, and kidney disease, with medication before they will admit their eating habits are causing their health issues. The cancer-come-and-get-me sign is fully illuminated above their head.

If you smoke, QUIT! Smoking cigarettes causes cancer. Electronic cigarettes are not a good substitute. The heating of the e-liquids converts into toxic compounds, according to the American Chemical Society.[1]

Drinking more soda than water in a day puts you in line for cancer. You are a likely candidate for cancer if you are consuming red meat two or more times a week because it is contaminated, difficult to digest, and is high in cholesterol. By now, you can see the patterns of health destruction. Cancer is directly related to what you put in your body. Unhealthy food means an unhealthy body. Healthy food means a healthy body. An unhealthy lifestyle means an unhealthy body. A healthy lifestyle means a healthy body.

I am not alone in knowing this information. There are many natural practitioners and medical doctors that know what you eat will determine your health status. Dr. Otto Heinrich Warburg received the Nobel Peace Prize in 1931 for discovering the cure for cancer. While some of his 1966 speech contains medical terminology that may be unfamiliar to you, please read every word. Dr. Warburg states that an acidic condition is the cause for cancer and that restoring the body to an alkaline state can inhibit the growth or existence of cancer.

The Prime Cause and Prevention of Cancer

Dr. Otto Warburg lecture delivered to Nobel Laureates on June 30, 1966, at Lindau, Lake Constance, Germany:

> *There are prime and secondary causes of diseases. For example, the prime cause of the plague is the plague bacillus, but secondary causes of the plague are filth, rats, and the fleas that transfer the plague bacillus from rats to man. By the prime cause of a disease, I mean one that is found in every case of the disease.*
>
> *Cancer, above all other diseases, has countless secondary causes. Almost anything can cause cancer. But, even for cancer, there is only one prime cause. The prime cause of cancer is the replacement of the respiration of oxygen (oxidation of sugar) in normal body cells by fermentation of sugar.*
>
> *All normal body cells meet their energy needs by respiration of oxygen, whereas cancer cells meet their energy needs in great part by fermentation. All normal body cells are thus obligate aerobes, whereas all cancer*

cells are partial anaerobes. From the standpoint of the physics and chemistry of life this difference between normal and cancer cells is so great that one can scarcely picture a greater difference. Oxygen gas, the donor of energy in plants and animals, is dethroned in the cancer cells and replaced by the energy yielding reaction of the lowest living forms, namely the fermentation of sugar. In every case, during the cancer development, the oxygen respiration always falls, fermentation appears, and the highly differentiated cells are transformed into fermenting anaerobes, which have lost all their body functions and retain only the now useless property of growth and replication. Thus, when respiration disappears, life does not disappear, but the meaning of life disappears, and what remains are growing machines that destroy the body in which they grow.

All carcinogens impair respiration directly or indirectly by deranging capillary circulation, a statement that is proven by the fact that no cancer cell exists without exhibiting impaired respiration. Of course, respiration cannot be repaired if it is impaired at the same time by a carcinogen. To prevent cancer it is therefore proposed first to keep the speed of the blood stream so high that the venous blood still contains sufficient oxygen; second, to keep high the concentration of hemoglobin in the blood; third, to add always to the food, even of healthy people, the active groups of the respiratory enzymes; and to increase the doses of these groups, if a precancerous state has already developed. If at the same time exogenous carcinogens are excluded rigorously, then much of the endogenous cancer may be prevented today.

These proposals are in no way utopian. On the contrary, they may be realized by everybody, everywhere, at any hour. Unlike the prevention of many other diseases, the prevention of cancer requires no government help, and not much money.

Many experts agree that one could prevent about 80% of all cancers in man, if one could keep away the known carcinogens from the normal body cells. But how can the remaining 20%, the so-called spontaneous cancers, be prevented? It is indisputable that all cancer could be prevented if the respiration of body cells were kept intact.

Nobody today can say that one does not know what the prime cause of cancer is. On the contrary, there is no disease whose prime cause is better known, so that today ignorance is no longer an excuse for avoiding measures for prevention. That the prevention of cancer will come there is no doubt. But how long prevention will be avoided depends on how long the prophets of agnosticism will succeed in inhibiting the application of scientific knowledge in the cancer field. In the meantime, millions of men and women must die of cancer unnecessarily.[2]

http://www.plasmafire.com/

Naturally Eradicating Cancer from Your Body

When you choose to eradicate cancer by flooding your body with nutrition, *there are no short-cuts.* Think of it this way. If a 35-foot wave is headed to shore, a 4-foot sandbag wall is not going to stop it. Eradicating cancer is the same way. You must eliminate all toxins and feed your body with organic, fresh, raw fruits and vegetables. Non-organic fruits and vegetables are not a substitute for organic. Non-organic produce contains pesticide and other contaminants that you will ingest. You must only drink alkaline water and organic tea.

No processed foods at all. No coffee. No animal products of any kind; not even organic. No alcohol. No cigarettes. No soda. No sugar. *No short-cuts!*

The real reason people do not eliminate cancer this way is because they are addicts. They are addicted to caffeine, sugar, yeast extract, bacon, alcohol, and cigarettes. They would rather die than change their eating habits.

The World Health Organization (WHO), through its cancer research agency, International Agency for Research on Cancer (IARC), provided the following information: "More than 30% of cancer deaths could be prevented by modifying or avoiding key risk factors, including:

- tobacco use
- being overweight or obese
- **unhealthy diet with low fruit and vegetable intake**
- lack of physical activity
- alcohol use
- sexually transmitted HPV-infection
- infection by HBV
- ionizing and non-ionizing radiation
- urban air pollution
- indoor smoke from household use of solid fuels."[3]

An unhealthy diet with low fruit and vegetable intake is number three on the list. Eating organic, fresh, raw fruits and vegetables is a strategy known throughout the world! In the United States, marketing a product is more important than the actual benefits of the product. Cancer is a multi-trillion dollar business. Why would any fast food chain want you to know that eating at its establishment will cause multiple health issues that will eventually drain your bank account and ultimately take your life entirely too early? They would not.

Your health will not hide your eating indiscretions. All those late-night cheeseburger binges and tequila shots eventually emerge from the darkness and into the light of the physician's office. You can smoke behind a building, drink until you pass out alone at home, chow down a container of ice cream in one sitting when no one is around, but eventually, the truth about your habits will come out. It will be disease.

You mean the world to someone. Your smile makes someone else's day. You have the ability to correct your bad habits and live and love a lot longer than the path you are on now.

The American Medical Association has these three options for you when you are diagnosed with cancer: surgery, radiation, or chemotherapy. These options are invasive, flood your already weakened body with chemicals and many times, they are often administered with less than a 20 percent chance of success.

"A short life is not given us, but we ourselves make it so."
–Seneca, AD 62

The medical community knows for a fact that the body can heal itself. So do you. When someone is operated on, everyone involved is fairly certain that the incision, blood vessels, tendons, nerves, and muscles will heal back together. If that was not the case, no one would elect to be operated on. It would, instead, be considered a crime, not a surgical procedure, if the body was not prone to healing back together.

For people involved in near-fatal motor vehicle collisions, the incidence of survival can be increased when the patient is placed in a coma until the body recovers to the point that natural movement will no longer endanger the person's life from severe injuries. Inducing a coma to allow serious trauma to heal is an acceptable practice in the United States.

I remember a curious practice from my youth when my mother's friend was going into the hospital for surgery. My mother announced that we had to go buy raisins immediately. We came home and she emptied the entire box into a mixing bowl and then poured water over the raisins making sure that the water was one inch above the top of the raisins.

When her friend got out of the hospital several days later, mother drained the water from the raisins into a quart jar and took it to her. The lady was supposed to drink the raisin water that day. Upon arriving home from her friend's house, my mother poured more water on the raisins to soak again overnight. She drained the water from the raisins again the next day and took it to her friend. I was confused about this practice until I began my education for natural health.

Raisins are among the most alkaline foods. Allowing the raisins to rehydrate in water for several days while her friend was in the hospital created an alkaline, super healing concoction to help counteract the negative effects of the toxic anesthesia, pain medications, and dehydration. Her friend drank the raisin water in lieu of food for three days. The fourth day, she ate some of the raisins.

The body is a healing machine when provided the right nutrition.

When you receive a cancer diagnosis, request a copy of your blood test. It should reveal your nutritional deficiency or imbalance. Cancer cannot live inside an alkaline body. Consult a doctor of natural medicine to assist you when you choose to handle your health issues with nutrition.

Vitamin supplements are not an acceptable replacement for fresh, raw organic fruits and vegetables. Pure vitamin C powder is the only exception.

"I firmly believe that if the whole materia medica could be sunk to the bottom of the sea, it would be better for mankind and all the worse for the fishes!"
–Dr. Oliver Wendell Holmes, 1879

Even in 1879 educated men knew that the doctor of medicine would not treat the cause, but only the symptoms. *Today, medical error is the fifth leading cause of death in the United States of America.* The majority of the medical errors are related to incorrect prescription medications.

Prescription medications and cancer treatment are too profitable for pharmaceutical companies, hospitals and medical doctors to ever endorse health through nutrition!

Have you traveled to any destination in the world with as many hospitals, cancer treatment centers, and specialty practices as there are in the United States? Well-traveled people can attest that most countries practice the principles to *"Let food be thy medicine and medicine be thy food."* This quote by Hippocrates, who is referred to as the "father of modern medicine," is what makes you well and keeps you well. We have all these medical buildings dedicated to health, when the reality is that they are built to aid in your health destruction. Economies are not fueled by keeping you healthy.

There is a distinct difference between requiring surgery after an accident to mend broken bones, remove foreign objects, and repair devastating wounds—and surgery to remove organs that can be restored through nutrition. The surgery after trauma is to save your life. The surgery to remove an organ can compromise your life.

After any surgery, a patient in a United States hospital, dedicated to health, is given soda, or diet soda if you have diabetes! Diet soda is served in hospitals! So is every kind of microwaved, unrecognizable piece of synthetic garbage disguised as food. After charging the extraordinary fees for a hospital stay, one would think they could at least afford to offer organic produce and some alkaline water!

The most prevalent questions when dealing with a cancer diagnosis is, “Where did it come from?” and “How did I get it?” All disease is caused by the same thing: too many toxins and not enough nutrition.

The medical community and pharmaceutical companies know the answer to cancer. There is no profit in telling you to quit eating junk and eat your organic fruits and vegetables and drink appropriate amounts of alkaline water. On top of that, most people would be extremely disappointed if their doctor told them to go home, keep all their money instead of an expensive and extensive hospital stay, give up all their favorite synthetic foods, drink water instead of beer or soda, rest, get some sunlight, and eat fresh organic fruits and vegetables, seeds and nuts, and you will be fine.

People have so much pride, they would rather take their chance with surgery and chemotherapy rather than admit they contributed to their own demise and just change their habits.

Knowing that one in three persons will receive a cancer diagnosis, what is your plan? You can spend your hard-earned money on synthetic foods that cause cancer and spend the

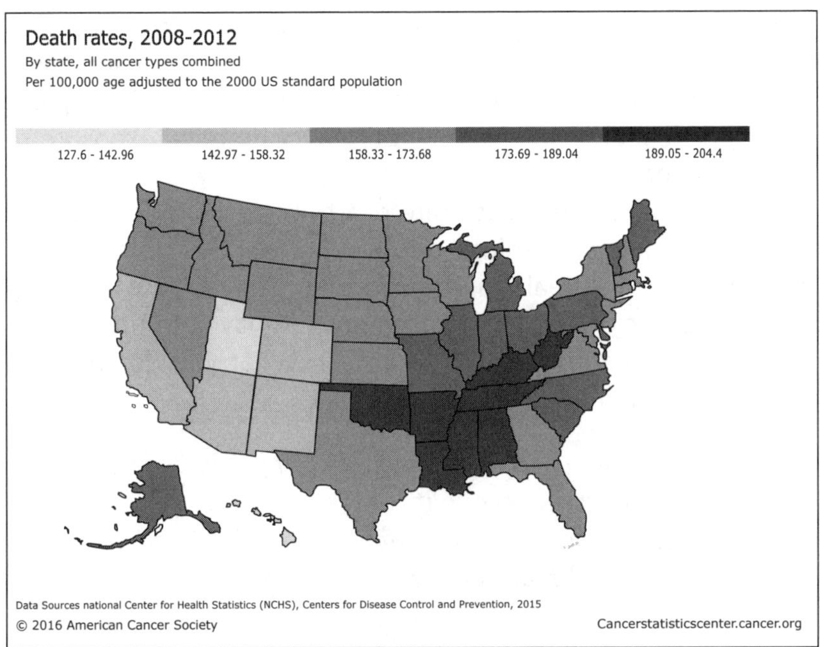
Death rates, 2008-2012
By state, all cancer types combined
Per 100,000 age adjusted to the 2000 US standard population
127.6 - 142.96
142.97 - 158.32
158.33 - 173.68
173.69 - 189.04
189.05 - 204.4
Data Sources national Center for Health Statistics (NCHS), Centers for Disease Control and Prevention, 2015
© 2016 American Cancer Society
Cancerstatisticscenter.cancer.org

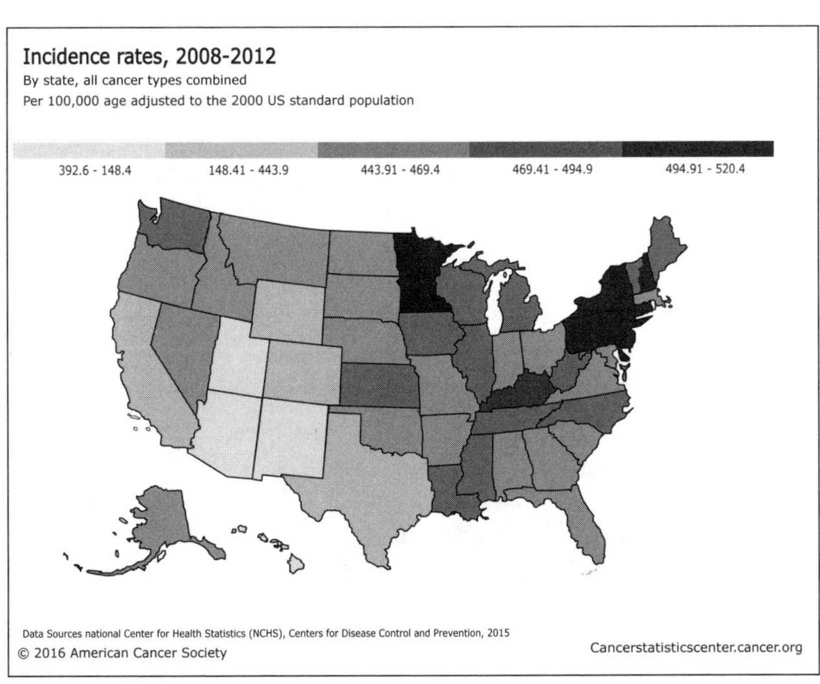
Incidence rates, 2008-2012
By state, all cancer types combined
Per 100,000 age adjusted to the 2000 US standard population
392.6 - 148.4
148.41 - 443.9
443.91 - 469.4
469.41 - 494.9
494.91 - 520.4
Data Sources national Center for Health Statistics (NCHS), Centers for Disease Control and Prevention, 2015
© 2016 American Cancer Society
Cancerstatisticscenter.cancer.org

remainder of your savings on the chemotherapy and/or radiation treatment that yields less than a 20 percent chance of success—or you can change your eating habits to include fresh, raw organic fruits and vegetables, and limit your environmental exposure to chemicals and toxins.

Viewing the cancer death rate chart, it is easy to identify the sweet tea, fried-everything Southern States. The states known for a more natural health approach and organic products show a lower incidence of cancer mortality. You now have the information you need to naturally eradicate cancer. What you do with this knowledge is up to you.

"The value you place on living a healthy existence with an uncompromised quality of life is the catalyst that will prompt change in your life. Death is final and good health does not come from a pill."

– DK Guyer, PhD

14

Crohn's Disease and Ulcerative Colitis

The Center for Disease Control (CDC) reports that the cause of ulcerative colitis and Crohn's disease are unknown. I know the cause. Hippocrates stated, "All disease begins in the gut." He knew the cause 2,000 years ago! Crohn's disease is the direct result of consuming food stuffs with little to no nutritional value. Since the body's cells are pre-programmed to stay alive, the cells in the intestine begin to attack other cells in the intestine searching for any amount of nutriment in order to stay alive.

Ulcerative colitis and Crohn's disease are the direct result of too many toxins and not enough nutrition. The reason all disease begins in the gut is because what we eat exits the body through the gut, the intestinal tract. Nutrient assimilation happens in the intestines. With the overconsumption of synthetic substances, contaminated meats and grains, excessive sugar, and little nutrition, the intestines cannot absorb any useful vitamins or minerals to sustain a healthy existence.

Anna's Story

This is the story of Anna—a senior in high school diagnosed with advanced Crohn's disease.

Anna's neighbor encouraged her to investigate some natural options before going through with her scheduled surgery to have a complete colectomy—removal of her intestines. She began her research online. After several hours of research and reading about natural remedies, Anna thought there may be an alternative to surgery. After reading six or seven articles to her mother, tears began to trickle down her face. She was distraught thinking about how this surgery would impact the remainder of her life.

Anna's mother located a naturopathic doctor and explained that her daughter had Crohn's disease to the extent that the surgeon was going to remove her bowel and that Anna would have a colostomy bag for the rest of her life. Prior to having her health begin to fail at an alarming rate, Anna was planning to go to college after graduation. She wanted to know if there was anything she could do to stop the operation and restore Anna's health.

The process began with questions about what Anna ate during the day. The answer was alarming, yet simple. Anna drank a diet soda while getting ready for school and did not eat breakfast. She ate pizza at lunch from the cafeteria at school with a diet soda and had french fries and another diet soda for dinner. She rarely drank water. She had been on her "diet" since the beginning of her sophomore year to lose weight. Although she had been to see a myriad of doctors and specialists, no one had ever questioned her eating habits.

The naturopathic doctor explained nutrition, water consumption, and why this was happening to Anna. Prior to her sophomore year, Anna liked fruits and vegetables and had eaten a varied diet. To start repairing the intestinal damage, Anna began a fruit and vegetable regimen starting out slowly with bananas, lettuce, watermelon, and broccoli, drinking water throughout the day, and Red Rooibos tea before bedtime. She added additional fruits and vegetables every two days. Her body was so nutrient deficient and her bowels so defunct that eating large amounts of anything would not have proved beneficial.

She had headaches and nausea from her body detoxifying, especially from the aspartame withdrawal associated with the diet soda consumption. After the first week, Anna was very weak and suffering occasional diarrhea and headaches but was eating fruits and vegetables. She stuck to the new regimen, increasing the variety of fresh fruits and vegetables as well as increasing her water consumption. By the end of the second week, the headaches began to subside. Anna began to have regular bowel movements. After four weeks, all the blotchy red patches on Anna's face had disappeared. She was eating full meals—breakfast, lunch, and dinner—using food combining methodology.

Anna's new diet not only restored her intestinal health, but saved her life as well. Had she gone through the surgery and returned to her diet soda, pizza, and french fry consumption for food, another type of disease would have most likely surfaced, further endangering her life.

The medical community diagnoses Crohn's disease and ulcerative colitis as a disease whereas the immune system mistakenly attacks the healthy bacteria in the intestines. This is not quite the case. The immune system is making no mistake! The immune system cannot function without nutrients. The only nutrients available are in the intestinal track. The intestines are where your food is assimilated into nutrients. When there are no nutrients being consumed, the cells search for nutriment within the other cells. It is not disease. It is the body trying to preserve its life. The body is in starvation mode. Even if the person with Crohn's disease is obese, they are still starving to death. Processed, synthetic, fast foods do not equate to nutrition. They equate to disease. The body never asks for food, only nutrition. Eating pounds and pounds of non-nutritious junk is the fastest way to a Crohn's disease and ulcerative colitis diagnosis.

If you know someone with Crohn's disease or ulcerative colitis, just watch what they eat for one day. After reading this book, you will be able to recognize why they are so sick. Encourage them to change their eating habits.

Crohn's disease is not a disease. You cannot catch it and you cannot inherit it. A Crohn's disease diagnosis reveals consistent consumption of contaminated and synthetic foodstuffs instead of healthy options. By drinking appropriate amounts of water, eating fresh, raw, organic fruits and vegetables, you can help eliminate intestinal complications and disease and restore your health.

"Breaking bad habits is not always easy. But if we don't break them, they will surely break us!"
—James Lennon, 1986

15

Diabetes

Diabetes is the fastest growing medical diagnosis in the United States. In this chapter, you will learn the cause of diabetes, why 95 percent of all diabetes diagnosis can be reversed without medication, and understand how to accomplish that goal.

Diabetes is considered a disease by the medical community because the body is not making enough insulin to accommodate the sugar in the blood (high blood sugar). During digestion, the body breaks down carbohydrates, starches, and sugars and produces glucose into the blood stream. Glucose is then absorbed into the cells for energy production. *Diabetes is not a disease.* It is the direct result of continually consuming more sugar than the body can process.

Many people believe that diabetes is based on family history and doctors advise patients that the propensity to become diabetic is genetic. I believe diabetes is related to family history, but not the family's genetics—it is the family's eating habits that are inherited.

Unless a conscious effort is made to do otherwise, Americans typically eat the same foods, prepared the same way that their parents and grandparents prepared them. If you were accustomed to meals of meat and potatoes growing up, it is what you learned to enjoy and prepare for your family.

The typical American Thanksgiving dinner is turkey, mashed potatoes, gravy, bread and butter, stuffing, corn, cranberry sauce, multiple pastry-type desserts, ice cream, sweet tea, and soda. Broken down into categories, it is contaminated protein, carbohydrates, starch, sugar, and fat. It is diabetes in the making.

American summer barbeques for Memorial Day, July Fourth celebrations, and Labor Day picnics include hot dogs, hamburgers, french fries, potato salad, noodle salads, corn on the cob, pies, ice cream, soda, candies, and a variety of alcohol beverages. Broken down into categories, it is a huge selection of health-destroying synthetic, contaminated food choices that lead to diabetes: contaminated protein, synthetic protein, starch, sugar, and more sugar, and little to no nutritional value. It is diabetes in the making.

With that said, many people are confused when it comes to making good choices. Maybe you are one of them. For example, one woman I met was so happy about her new healthy food choices that when she went on a date at a local chain restaurant, she chose the spinach and artichoke dip instead of cheese sticks for an appetizer. She was so pleased with her healthy decision. It sounds like a better option, but the facts say differently.

	Artichoke & Spinach Dip	***Cheese Sticks***
Fat	94 g	48 g
Cholesterol	not listed	not listed
Carbohydrates	84 g	111 g
Sodium	2640 g	2680 g
Protein	43 g	29 g

Which one looks like a better option to you? If you answered neither, you are well on your way to making healthier choices! Remember that this is just the appetizer—the main course has not yet arrived!

We view food as *"What are you in the mood for?"* when making choices instead of asking *"What nutrients does my body need?"* Where does natural vitamin C come from? Cheese sticks is not the correct answer, but some people do not know the answer and they do not know exactly what is in the food they are consuming.

When purchasing so-called food at the grocery store, many choose options they like instead of options that provide vitamins, minerals, and natural sources of fiber. Somewhere along the way grapefruits and oranges, blueberries, peaches, plums, and carrots have been replaced with chips and pretzels, artificial fruit juice and gourmet coffees with synthetic creamer. The best way to understand what you are consuming and the dangers lurking behind the "researched marketing" on the package is to read the label.

I estimate that one standard American meal contains more carbohydrates, starch, sugar, and chemicals than is ingested in most countries in a week! And that is only one meal, not three meals a day.

If you have to take a pill every day, where is the cure? A cure means you are cured and there would be no need to continue to take the medication. The pill only masks the destruction of your body when people on diabetes medications continue to ignore the rules of digestion and continually consume carbohydrates and sugar. Being diagnosed with diabetes is like having the "check engine" light come on in your vehicle and stay on. The longer you ignore the warning, the fewer days you have until the vehicle (your body) just won't operate anymore.

Let's start at the beginning and take a look at how diabetes initiates and the influence your medical doctor has on the progression of your diabetes diagnosis.

1. You are led to believe that there is something wrong with your body because it cannot produce the correct amount of insulin to accommodate your sugar intake.
2. You are not informed that the eating habits you have been taught could be contributing to the condition; rather, an inherited gene is explained as the culprit for your disease.
3. You are then scheduled to meet with a dietician and are instructed to consume protein with every meal and count your carbohydrate consumption.
4. The dietician does not explain the nutritional difference when consuming a banana as a carbohydrate versus eating a sweet roll as a carbohydrate. Eating protein with every meal disallows the proper digestion and assimilation of

other valuable nutrients and floods the body with toxins from contaminated meats and farm-raised fish.

5. You are prescribed medication to manage your disease with no apparent hope of ever returning to good health.
6. In respect to your declining health, you are advised to self-check your sugar daily and have an institutional blood analysis performed routinely to determine if the prescription medication is affecting your kidney or liver function.
7. At no time in this process are you provided any factual information that will allow you to consume a natural diet and eliminate the symptoms of diabetes entirely so you can live without prescription medication dependence.

This list describes the steps in place for pharmaceutical companies and the medical community to exploit the condition known as diabetes by taking advantage of the general populations' lack of real nutrition education and creates an environment for people to believe that they truly have a disease.

Since only 5 percent of all diabetes cannot be reversed through diet changes, that means the remaining 95 percent of all diagnosed diabetics can become non-diabetic by changing their diet.

Eliminating all synthetic, processed foods is the first step to regaining your health. Eating contaminated protein with every meal will not provide the vitamins and minerals needed for proper body function.

Carbohydrates, starches, and sugars are not created equal and they are the food category that is least understood. Learning about how sugar processes in your body will help you make educated choices.

Refined White Sugar

First, refined white sugar is a foreign substance to your body. In its natural form, sugar is not white. The natural whole food components that allow your body to process real sugar cane are removed from refined white sugar. Calcium hydroxide, sulfur dioxide, bleaching agents and other chemicals are used to further process the sugar. The end result is pure sucrose, which requires higher levels of insulin production within the body to convert the refined white sugar into glucose.

When consuming fruit, the body's insulin production can handle and more easily convert the whole food sugars, in their natural state, into glucose. Many diabetics are warned against consuming fruit. The body can handle assimilating fruit sugars faster and easier than any other sugar to glucose conversion. Fruit sugars are whole and more easily digested sugars.

Refined white sugar is a chemically altered substance that creates addiction. In lab rats given the option between cocaine and sugar, the rats chose sugar even after they had tried the highly addictive cocaine! *Ninety-five percent of all diagnosed diabetics can change their health status to non-diabetic in sixty to ninety days by changing their diet.*

Bread

Since the carbohydrates category encompasses a large variety of foods, let's examine the most consumed, highly-processed carbohydrate—bread.

The USDA National Nutrient Database states that one slice of white bread has 1.4 grams of sugar. With that information, two slices of white bread to make a sandwich would contain just over one half teaspoon of sugar. That does not seem too horrible until you consider that the half teaspoon of sugar only accounts for the bread and does not include the carbohydrate content, which is a whooping 25 grams before anything is placed between the slices.

Carbohydrates turn into glucose (blood sugar) during digestion. What that means is those 25 grams have now become a little over six teaspoons of sugar metabolizing directly into the blood stream. This is the reason why athletes will often ingest carbohydrates (bananas and oranges, for example) for energy. The conversion from food into glucose occurs very quickly producing a sustainable amount of energy.

Bread digests in the body as sugar, yeast, and glucose (carbohydrates). In actuality, two slices of bread equates to more than 6 teaspoons of sugar in the body. Bread is not a recommended substance for a diabetic.

Do the Math

There are so many products on the grocery shelves being marketed as healthy and low in sugar, but the math tells the truth. Always read the label and do the math. Remember, 1 teaspoon of sugar equals 4 grams. Here's how it works:

One individual serving cup of fruited yogurt equals 25 grams of sugar.

How to do the math: 25 g sugar divided by 4 equals 6.25 teaspoons sugar (grams of sugar / 4 = teaspoons of sugar). Here, the number 4 is used as a constant for conversion.

Total carbohydrates use the same calculation: Grams of the total carbs divided by 4 equals the teaspoons of sugar that would metabolize into glucose.

Double cheeseburger (50 g), medium french fries (53 g), 16 oz. chocolate shake (131 g)

How to do the math: Add the total carbohydrates: 50 g + 53 g + 131 g = 234 g

Now use the same equation as before: 234 g divided by 4 equals 58.5 teaspoons sugar

This meal contains almost ten times the amount of sugar recommended per day by the World Health Organization! Nice lunch, huh? If you eat this way regularly, you are either diabetic or having undiagnosed health issues.

The World Health Organization recommends ***6 teaspoons of sugar per day.*** Diabetes is killing men, women, children, and fetuses all around the globe due to processed food products with high sugar content. Excessive sugar equates to cellular destruction!

Because the ingredient labels list carbohydrates and sugar in grams, many Americans do not comprehend the amount of sugar because it is not stated in ounces or teaspoons. For example: 16 grams of sugar seems miniscule compared to reading 4 teaspoons of sugar per serving on a label. Add to this the fact that rarely do Americans consume a serving size of anything! A serving size of ice cream is half a cup, not half of the container. A serving size of soda contains 42 grams of sugar and is 12 fluid ounces, not half of the 2-liter bottle.

Read the Labels

Reading labels and understanding that 4 grams of sugar or carbohydrates equates to one teaspoon of sugar may help keep things in perspective. Refined white sugar also contains chemicals, which are toxic substances the body has to process and expel, creating another reason to limit sugar intake.

An additional complication of diabetes is candida yeast. Let me explain. Candida is an incredible warrior inside the body, defending it from the dangers of excessive sugar. Candida rises to eat the sugar in your body in order to save your life. The problem occurs when excessive sugar consumption occurs over and over again. The candida response to the extraordinary amount of sugar intake becomes overwhelming. Candida yeast accumulates in the intestinal tract and inhibits the assimilation of nutrients. In some diabetics, the candida yeast accumulation in the bowel is so extreme, it forms a barrier between the actual intestinal wall and the digested food traveling through the intestines so nutrient extraction and assimilation cannot occur at all!

Limiting the amount of carbohydrate and sugar consumption limits the production of candida. Supplementing your diet with a high-quality probiotic can also reduce the negative effects of candida. Hippocrates's statement deserves repeating, *"All disease begins in the gut."* Keeping candida under control helps you maintain a healthy gut.

For 95 percent of those diagnosed with diabetes, there is hope. When you alter your diet by reducing dangerous carbohydrates and sugars, providing your body with vital nutrients to fortify your cells instead of destroying them, you are establishing a foundation for better health.

I have heard the saying when people perish from the complications of diabetes that they lost the battle to the disease. The reality is that they were never given the tools to fight the battle. They were instructed to eat protein with every meal, count synthetic carbohydrates, avoid fruit filled with nutrition, and prescribed a lifetime of prescription medication. They were uninformed and mislead. Their diabetes education established an inability to provide their body with the nutritional requirements to become healthy. Instead of eating endless amounts of destructive, processed sweet delights, and prescription medications, they could have opted for nutritious choices and lived a longer, healthier, wealthier existence with the proper education.

It is time to change the way we perceive food and eating. We should eat to live. Not live to eat whatever, whenever, and any amount we desire. Help the ones you love regain their lively health through nutrition and correct nutrition information.

16

Fibromyalgia

Let's get right down to the published facts from the medical community addressing fibromyalgia.

Fibromyalgia is defined as a disorder described by unexplained widespread pain, with fatigue, sleep disorders, memory loss, and issues associated with depression and anxiety. Fibromyalgia is believed to be overactive nerves responsible for the pain. The encompassing pain causes fatigue, inability to obtain proper rest and sleep, brain fog, and headaches.

There is no known cause or cure for the affliction known as fibromyalgia by the medical community. Persons with fibromyalgia symptoms are diagnosed and prescribed medications for the condition based solely on reported symptoms. There is no test to determine that you have fibromyalgia.

Fibromyalgia pain is *real.* The person being diagnosed with fibromyalgia symptoms is feeling the pain. I do not discredit the patient's symptoms diagnosed as fibromyalgia. The symptoms are real; however, it is not a disease and it is not inherited. Fibromyalgia is the result of too many toxins and not enough nutrition.

Many people who are diagnosed with fibromyalgia are already being treated with prescription medications for tension headaches, anxiety, depression, post-traumatic stress disorder, and irritable bowel syndrome.

Antianxiety and antidepressant medications list the following common side effects:[1]

- Upset stomach, constipation, diarrhea
- Fatigue, weakness
- Headache
- Memory problems, confusion, trouble concentrating
- Insomnia, sleeplessness
- Nervousness
- Dizziness, blurred vision

Strangely, these side effects replicate the fatigue, sleep disorders, headaches, pain or cramping in the lower abdomen and cognitive difficulties described as symptoms of fibromyalgia.

Fibromyalgia is an umbrella disease category to place patients under because it is more preferable to prescribe medications that reduce the pain while the destruction of the body continues.

Lyrica, the most common drug prescribed for fibromyalgia symptoms, has side effects as well. The more common side effects of Lyrica[2] are:

- accidental injury
- bloating or swelling of the face, arms, hands, lower legs, or feet
- blurred vision
- **burning, tingling, numbness or pain in the hands, arms, feet, or legs**
- change in walking and balance
- clumsiness
- **confusion**
- **delusions**
- **dementia**
- **difficulty having a bowel movement (stool)**
- difficulty with speaking
- double vision
- dry mouth
- fever
- **headache**

- hoarseness
- increased appetite
- lack of coordination
- **loss of memory**
- **lower back or side pain**
- painful or difficult urination
- **problems with memory**
- **rapid weight gain**
- **seeing double**
- **sensation of pins and needles**
- shakiness and unsteady walk
- **sleepiness or unusual drowsiness**
- **stabbing pain**
- swelling
- **tingling of the hands or feet**
- trembling, or other problems with muscle control or coordination
- unusual weight gain or loss

For someone already experiencing unexplained pain, headaches, brain fog, sleep disorders, depression, anxiety, and post-traumatic stress disorder, this option does not appear to be viable. The side effects listed are the more common side effects. Less common side effects are not listed.

Fibromyalgia, as a disease, should be listed as caused by the over consumption of toxic materials marketed as "safe" to unsuspecting, loving, kind, amazing, trusting people.

The pain of the fibromyalgia symptoms can be debilitating. It is not a medical issue that is causing the pain. The body is riddled with toxins, and in many cases, is the direct result of side effects of other prescription medications.

A diet including organic green tea and an abundant consumption of antioxidant-rich organic fresh fruits and vegetables can provide the much-needed nutrients required to naturally begin healing compromised cells.

Here is how the majority of the fibromyalgia symptoms can be eliminated. Please keep in mind, medication is being prescribed for a condition based solely on symptoms, not the cause.

1. Eliminate all processed foods.
2. Drink only alkaline water (at least six glasses per day) and 3 to 4 cups of certified organic green tea.
3. As your body is detoxifying, your pain may increase. Each cell in your body will be expelling toxins. Imagine that it is equivalent to mini-surgeries throughout all your tissues to restore your health.
4. Rest.
5. Get some sunshine for at least twenty minutes a day. A real source of vitamin D will help you feel better.
6. Eat only fresh, raw organic fruits and vegetables.

The reason people remain sick is because eating healthy fruits and vegetables is not all that appealing to them. Toxic foodstuffs are laced with synthetic components to create an addiction to their taste. Autolyzed yeast extract is considered to be as addictive as heroine. Making the change to eating nutritious foods is difficult. When people do not have the energy to get up and get a shower due to the symptoms of fibromyalgia, changing their eating habits may seem impossible.

It can be done, but it may require help from friends, family, neighbors and coworkers. Returning to a healthy life is important. People are willing to help; they simply need to be asked for their assistance.

17

Heart Disease

Heart disease is the number one killer in the United States. A modified diet is the fastest, easiest way to reverse heart disease before it is too late. People can survive without an appendix, but not without a functioning heart. It is a priceless asset that protects your life.

The one health condition that nearly everyone in the natural health and medical communities can agree on when it comes to both the cause and remedy is heart disease. Unless you are born with a severe heart condition, nearly all cardiovascular disease is caused by eating habits and lifestyle.

According to the World Health Organization, there are steps that can be taken to reduce cardiovascular diseases worldwide:[1]

Examples of population-wide interventions that can be implemented to reduce CVDs include:

- *Comprehensive tobacco control policies*
- *Taxation to reduce the intake of foods that are high in fat, sugar, and salt*
- *Building walking and cycle paths to increase physical activity*
- *Strategies to reduce harmful use of alcohol*
- *Providing healthy school meals to children*

Reducing cardiovascular disease risks is a short list, but abiding by the rules is not as easy for some people. Exercise, monitor your sugar, salt, and fat intake, do not drink alcohol in excess, do not smoke tobacco, do not use e-cigarettes, avoid processed foods, drink appropriate amounts of water, and consume a healthy diet of fresh, raw, highly nutritional fruits and vegetables.

For the majority of people suffering from heart disease, it simply comes down to education. Believe it or not, heart disease is rarely inherited. Eating habits, however, are often passed down to each generation.

Here is the quickest, easiest way to make healthy heart choices—if it is not found in nature, do ***not*** *eat it.*

There are no bacon double cheeseburgers in nature. They are one of the most disastrous heart health food items because they are normally consumed with french fries and a large soda. Chicken Alfredo with garlic bread is a heart attack on a plate. Pizza with a variety of meats and meat substitutes is horrific for heart health.

Every day and with each bite you take, you are determining your future health.

One small hamburger once a month does not cause the same damage as eating double cheeseburgers for lunch every day. The more often you consume processed, high sugar, high cholesterol meals, the faster cardiovascular disease surfaces.

Heart disease does not develop overnight. It is a compilation of years of ingesting poor food choices. By addressing cardiovascular issues early and modifying your diet, hypertension and cholesterol can be halted for many years.

High blood pressure is described as the silent killer. It is the result of consuming too much sodium and high fat foods and not enough water to achieve a proper balance.

Sodium nitrates contained in processed or packaged foods are not a real source of sodium. They are synthetic and can exacerbate hypertension. Real sodium comes from sea salt and certain vegetables. Everyone needs a minimum of 1,800-2,000 mg of sodium daily when drinking five to six (8 ounce) glasses of water and experiencing normal mobility. If you ingest a high sodium diet, you will need to drink much more water to stabilize your blood pressure than someone who monitors their sodium intake.

Cholesterol and arterial plaque is the direct result of ingesting too many high cholesterol foods and not enough cholesterol-reducing foods. Unless their life is threatened with debilitating stroke or even death, rarely does anyone monitor their cholesterol consumption. They prefer to pop a pill and hope that it helps. Only by modifying your diet can you limit the continuing destruction of your heart and arteries. Processed and synthetic foods are a guaranteed way to destroy your health.

Taking prescription medications to control hypertension in lieu of modifying your diet creates accompanying health conditions. It does not remove the damage being caused by high blood pressure conditions.

Medications, over time, place a strain on all the organs, especially the kidneys. Medications are synthetic compounds and often cause dehydration. Hypertension medications cause more frequent urination and the result, even if you are diligent about drinking appropriate amounts of water, is dehydration.

Not only do the kidneys have to accommodate the diuretic effects of the medication, the tissues in the kidneys are consistently exposed to the toxic waste created by the medication.

The most effective way of protecting your cardiovascular health is eating fresh, raw organic fruits and vegetables. Contrary to popular belief, a high-protein diet does not protect your heart or any other organ. A high-protein diet is a certain path to heart disease because meats in the United States are contaminated with dangerous chemicals and they are inherently higher in fat and cholesterol.

Your foods choices either encourage great health or prompt disease. You are in complete control of your heart health. Exercise, appropriate water consumption, and monitoring your cholesterol and sodium intake are your responsibilities. The resulting condition of your level of heart disease is directly a result of your eating habits.

In this diagram, the first artery shown has a healthy flow of blood. As high cholesterol foods are consumed, plaque builds along the artery walls inhibiting the appropriate transport of blood. Eventually, as plague accumulates, the artery becomes impassable, limiting life-sustaining flow of blood.[2]

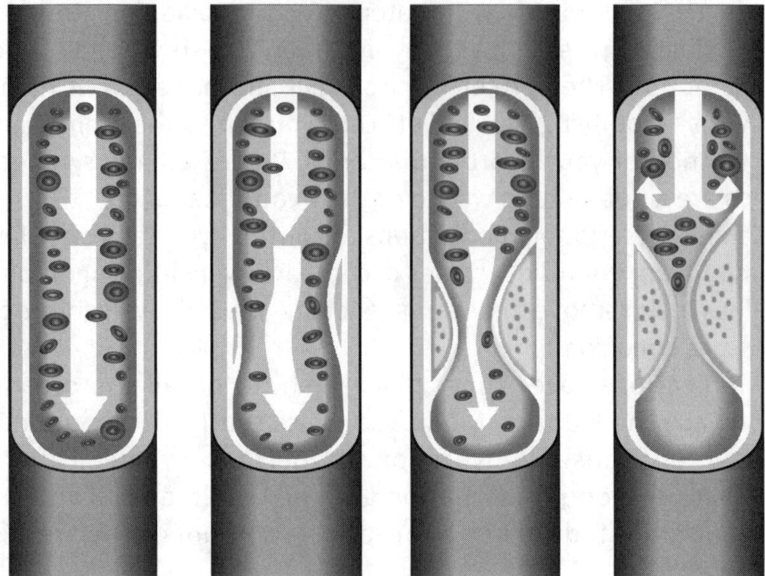

The following graphic by the CDC reveals the heart disease death rates in the United States.[3]

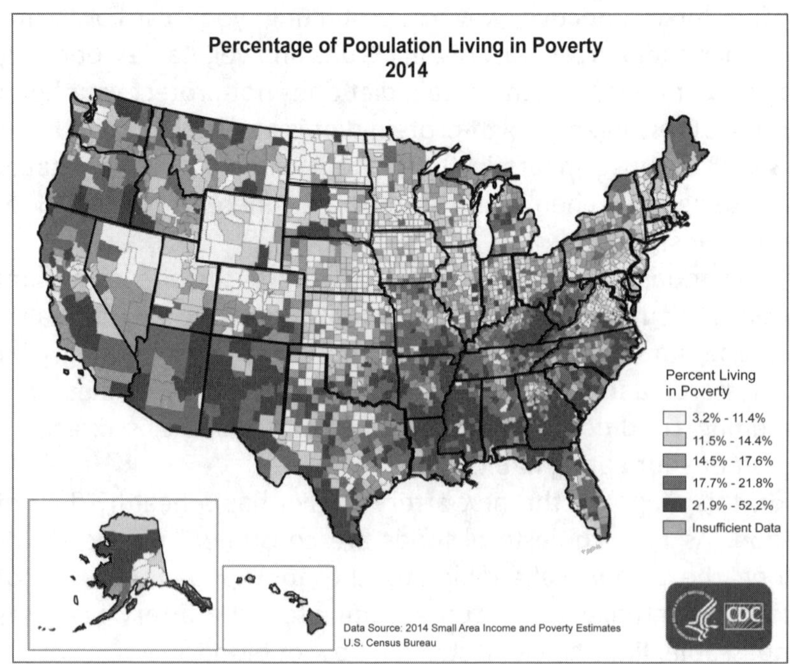

18

Kidney Disease

Your kidneys perform an incredible job of removing excess fluid and waste from your blood. They also release three important hormones:

1. Erythropoietin, crucial for making red blood cells.
2. Renin, essential for regulating blood pressure.
3. The active form of vitamin D, fundamental for maintaining calcium and normal chemical balance in the body.[1]

Most people are unaware of the incredibly important functions the kidneys perform. Treating your kidneys with ultimate respect will help keep you healthy. In order to limit kidney damage, let's look at what causes it.

Severe dehydration is a widespread condition affecting people of every age. Exchanging soda, coffee, energy drinks, flavored waters, sweet tea, juices, beer or wine in place of drinking plain alkaline water attributes to severe dehydration. There is no replacement for pure water for good health. Following the guidelines for water consumption printed in this book will help flush deadly toxins from your body, especially the kidneys, and will keep you hydrated.

Acidic food consumption wreaks havoc on the kidneys. The PRAL list (Potential Renal Acid Load) is an incredible source of information for the person suffering kidney disease at any level. We have already discussed that no disease can exist in an alkaline body and that all disease is caused by the same thing—too many toxins and not enough nutrition.

When consuming 80 percent of your daily calories in alkaline foods and 20 percent in acidic foods, you drastically improve the functions of your kidneys. The alkaline foods are predominately fresh, raw fruits and vegetables. They provide abundant nutrients and have hydrating juices. There is an obvious difference between eating a serving of fresh watermelon or a bakery item. The natural juices in the watermelon provide hydration and are an alkaline food. The bakery item creates dehydration and is acidic foodstuff. Following the 80/20 alkaline/acidic consumption rule can help eradicate kidney disease.

Prescription medications can cause kidney damage. The list is phenomenal. Medications prescribed for the following health complaints can be detrimental. The following are just a few of the medications that can attribute to kidney disease.

Acid reflux	Anesthetics	Anxiety
Antibiotics	Arthritis	Blood pressure
Cancer	Chemotherapy	Cholesterol
Chronic Fatigue	Constipation	Cystic fibrosis
Depression	Diabetes	Eczema
Fertility	Grave's disease	Heart disease
Heartburn	HIV	Hypertension
Impotence	Irritable Bowel (IBS)	Kidney stones
Malaria	Migraines	Mental illness
Multiple sclerosis	Muscular dystrophy	Pain killers
Parkinson's Disease	Rheumatoid Arthritis	Seizures
Sleep disorders	Stomach Ulcers	Thyroid

Most of the time, the medication is prescribed with the belief that the benefits will outweigh the negative side effects. The negative side effects create an ailment that will generate the opportunity for another prescription medication to be prescribed.

Over-the-counter pain relievers, cough, cold and flu relief, laxatives, nausea and diarrhea relief, allergy relief, and a variety of other medications also limit kidney function when these products are used on a consistent basis.

If you are currently taking a medication that requires blood tests to check your kidney function, you may want to consider finding a more natural way of handling your health situation and make it a priority.

Alcohol and illegal drug abuse, smoking and electronic cigarettes pose direct threats to your kidney function. There is an incorrect mindset that if your grandfather smoked and drank every day and lived into his late 70s, that all the warnings about this lifestyle are nonsense.

Over the past 50 years, the chemical additives to cigarettes and alcohol production has been extensive. A cigarette in the 1970s smelled sweet and was made of mainly tobacco. A cigarette today contains approximately 600 chemicals and the smell is not so sweet.

Beer, wine, and spirits are not produced the same way either. They are commercially produced with GMO grains, refined sugars, pesticide-laden fruits, artificial ingredients, and added synthetics.

Having a few cocktails today is more like having a few synthetic cocktails with a side of kidney disease. Alcohol always promotes severe dehydration. Illegal drug use subjects every part of the body to disease. Electronic cigarettes are chemicals.

Refined sugar promotes kidney disease. Drinking soda daily diminishes the ability of the kidneys to process excess waste in the blood. One 12-ounce serving of soda contains 42 g of sugar, which equates to just over 10 teaspoons of sugar in the blood. The World Health Organization recommends 6 teaspoons of sugar per day. Excessive consumption of baked goods, breads, frozen desserts, fruited yogurts, salty snacks, and candies, for example, promote kidney disease.

Kidney stones are a clear indication that the kidneys are compromised, and without a diet change, more extensive kidney disease complications are on the horizon. It is the common belief that some people just naturally have more uric acid, and kidney stones are an anomaly they have to accept. It is not a true conclusion. The acidic load on the kidneys is a direct result of the foods and drinks consumed. Kidney stones are common with heavy meat, bread, alcohol, and yeast product consumption.

Dark or foul-smelling urine tells the story. Proper hydration and nutritional food consumption creates clear or very near to clear urine. Dark urine screams dehydration and impending kidney disease! Eliminate this situation immediately by drinking pure alkaline water to help flush waste from your body in a more effective manner. Eliminate processed sugars and processed foods.

The kidneys are crucial organs responsible for clearing waste from your blood and eliminating extra fluid. Kidney function is extremely important for health at any level and kidney disease announces itself in advance of total disaster.

Preventing kidney disease begins with following nature's protocol for great health. Eating fresh, raw organic fruits and vegetables, drinking alkaline water, and eliminating contamination of the body by removing chemicals and synthetic products from daily consumption help protect the body from chronic kidney disease. When you correct your diet, you can restore kidney function over time. It is not an overnight process. It took time to accumulate the damage and it will take time to recover the damage.

19

Lyme Disease

Lyme disease is defined as the reaction in the body to parasites known as spirochetes that are a result of a bite from an infected deer tick. People diagnosed with Lyme disease often have no credible test results to support their diagnosis. According to the Centers for Disease Control and Prevention, there are no current testing platforms for Lyme disease that are deemed accurate.

The current treatment for Lyme disease is an extraordinary regimen of antibiotic prescriptions lasting for months and even years. Needless to say, this is not an acceptable treatment for any human being. It is extremely destructive.

Extended daily use of antibiotics creates antibiotic-resistant parasites within the body. In other words, if the first round of antibiotics did not kill the parasites, the second and third and fourth rounds of antibiotics will not kill them either; the excessive treatment renders any remaining parasites resistant to the antibiotics. This is true for all the parasites in the body, not just spirochetes.

Let's examine some of the dangers associated with back to back antibiotic prescriptions and why so many people diagnosed with Lyme rarely see any improvement.

The first alarming observation I've noticed is that many physicians who are self-proclaimed Lyme disease experts do not accept health insurance. A medical doctor claiming to be an expert, in any field, who does not accept any form of health insurance should immediately raise a red flag for concern about the validity of their practice. In addition, the majority of these physicians only accept cash. If their practice and intentions were in your best interest, you would be accepted under health insurance (yes, health insurance companies do cover some of the treatment for Lyme) for the office visit, the resulting prescription medication, and your health record would identify your condition.

These scam artists run under the radar, so to speak, taking advantage of many people by taking their money, destroying their health, and compromising their future and the future of their family.

Another very scary situation is knowing that you have never been bitten by a tick, especially one that created a bullseye reaction, and yet you are receiving a Lyme disease diagnosis. In other words, you should not be treated for a snake bite, if you have not been bitten by a snake. To clear up another myth, you cannot contract Lyme disease through salvia or sexual contact.

The fatigue, restlessness, pain and muscle weakness a patient feels is *real.* People being diagnosed with Lyme disease are truly experiencing these issues. They are also, however, experiencing symptoms of acidosis. Most are not experiencing Lyme disease. The first prescription of antibiotics, over the course of fourteen days, would have killed the parasites if there was a questionable tick bite. All additional antibiotics riddle the body with toxins, cause excessive yeast in the intestinal tract by destroying the good bacteria that aids in nutrient extraction, and the end result is the continued decline of the person's health. The bottom line is this—continued antibiotic treatment destroys your natural immune system. In addition, due to the destruction of the good bacteria in the bowels, the person essentially begins to starve to death because nutrient extraction is severely limited.

In order to offset the destruction of antibiotics in the intestinal tract, persons are advised to use probiotics. Taking one probiotic daily to combat an antibiotic prescription of 1,000 mg to help restore intestinal health is equivalent in effectiveness to putting two drops of water on a mud-covered windshield in order to clean it off. Probiotics need to be taken multiple times throughout the day in order to achieve any positive outcome.

Lyme disease testing is, to this day, not a proven science. According to a recent report from the Centers for Disease

Control (CDC), there is no benefit to prolonged antibiotic use for managing Lyme disease. Furthermore, there are no studies at all, ever, anywhere on the earth that conclude antibiotic treatment for Lyme disease is effective and should prevail longer than fourteen days.

The CDC is responsible for ensuring the safety of consumers. You may have seen and read the signs that are routinely displayed in medical offices stating that antibiotics are not prescribed for viral infections such as cold and flu symptoms. This practice is in place in order to reduce the prevalence of antibiotic-resistance bacteria known as super bugs.

Consider the treatment for a deadly form of MRSA (Methicillin, resistant Staphylococcus aureus) infection, a bacterial infection that can kill you within days if it enters your blood stream. It is treated with an antibiotic cocktail of three different antibiotics for fourteen days. Lyme disease is not a killer. Many people relinquish themselves to months of antibiotic treatment and are not absolved of the supposed condition.

Most people believe they have Lyme disease, even those who have never been bitten by a tick, have never walked through the woods, a field, or even across a grassy knoll, because a medical doctor told them they had symptoms of Lyme disease.

Treatment for Lyme disease is a complicated mess, to say the least. A Lyme disease diagnosis is so alarming and yet the treatment is unsuccessful because it does not include the nutrition factor.

Herbal treatments for Lyme disease help ease symptoms for these reasons. The herbal treatments help the body eliminate toxins, help fortify the weakened immune system and strengthen cells.

That being said, these treatments are only a small portion of trying to restore health. Without eliminating the toxic prescription medications, drinking appropriate amounts of water, and ingesting organic, fresh, raw fruits and vegetables for nutrition, the *symptoms* of the Lyme disease diagnosis will remain. The symptoms are a result of an acidic, toxic diet.

People diagnosed with Lyme disease are adamant that they have the affliction. Unfortunately, they are victims being treated for symptoms, not the actual cause. They remain on antibiotics, and in addition, some are prescribed malaria medication for the presence of babesia, another type of parasite. Babesiosis surfaces as flu-like conditions in elderly persons and unhealthy individuals with compromised immune function. Babesiosis rarely affects healthy people even if it can be identified in their blood.

When the cause, acidosis, is treated, the symptoms subside and health can be restored with continued consumption of whole, natural forms of nutrition.

20

Migraines and Headaches

Migraines and headaches are symptoms the body utilizes to create a sense of urgency for the problem that exists. As stated in Chapter 15 about diabetes, think of a headache or a migraine as your body's way of illuminating a "check engine" light. An automobile is set up with lights that appear on the dashboard to visibly remind the operator that the automobile requires maintenance or fluids to keep it functioning—the body has its own version of warning signals.

Migraines and headaches are rarely viewed as an alert or alarm of an underlying situation. Headaches are treated with an over-the-counter pain reliever and persistent migraines are usually addressed with prescription medications.

The cause of an intermittent headache is most likely apparent. When experiencing a headache while suffering a sinus infection or congestion, it is relatively easy to understand that a headache can occur do to impaired breathing (getting enough oxygen to the brain) or restricted blood flow due to inflamed sinus membranes and the sinus pressure that results.

A hangover headache from drinking too much alcohol is fairly self-explanatory—severe dehydration and too many toxins.

When sitting in a vehicle, with arms outstretched on the steering wheel and looking straight ahead for countless hours on a long trip, many drivers experience a tension headache due to minimal mobility, dehydration, and stressful driving encounters. The headache will persist after the driver has reached the destination and until the muscles in the neck and shoulder regions become relaxed, the stress factors are removed, and the body is rehydrated.

These types of headaches are very common and the cause is quickly identified and remedied and life goes on. I equate these types of headaches to the oil light on the dashboard. After the oil is added or changed, the light goes out.

But what happens when headaches are occurring and the cause is not easily identified? The most predominant causes of migraines or headaches are:

- Severe dehydration
- Reaction to a food additive or medication
- Head or neck injury

Delving into the details surrounding these causes will provide information for subsiding or eliminating migraines and headaches.

Severe Dehydration

Migraine headaches can only be described as excruciating pain. The onset of migraine headaches has many people confused about what causes them and how to stop their occurrence. Migraine headaches occur when blood flow becomes restricted due to dehydration or caffeine, loss of vitamins and minerals, and/or low oxygen in the blood. When dehydration is recognized as the headache arrives, it is often too late to arrest a full-blown migraine because the body cannot be rehydrated instantaneously. To avoid dehydration headaches of any severity, practice drinking at least 8 ounces of alkaline water every one to two hours throughout the day. Drinking water is an easy step to take in order to eliminate the horrific pain associated with a dehydration migraine.

Soda and coffee are not replacements for water. Some people are under the very dangerous assumption that as long as you are consuming liquids, it counts as water because it is made of water. *This is not a true assumption.* Pure alkaline water provides hydration. The caffeine, sugar, and artificial colors and flavors in soda and coffee act as diuretics and restrict blood flow causing dehydration.

There is no substitute for pure water. In a study by the CDC, less than 43 percent of the US population drinks four cups or more of water a day.[1] Dehydration is an epidemic that creates many health issues but can be easily eradicated by drinking water. Staying hydrated helps eliminate the onset of headaches and chronic migraines.

I have heard many accounts from people suffering migraine headaches. A wonderful woman was shopping in the retail store when she overheard another customer inquiring about a natural remedy for migraines for her daughter in college. The following is the story the woman shared about her own daughter.

Her very athletic and extremely health-conscious daughter began suffering migraines during her second semester in college her freshman year. While migraines are an accepted ailment for college students due to late study hours, more caffeinated product consumption, lack of sleep, and change in diet, her mother became very concerned. The young lady, we will name Victoria, was missing classes due to the intense migraines.

Victoria went to see a specialist. He prescribed an anti-seizure medication for her migraines. Her health began to deteriorate at a rapid rate after taking the medication the first week. After reading all the side effects of the medication and learning that stopping the medication without being weaned off of it could cause additional health complications, she took Victoria back to see the specialist. He insisted that Victoria was experiencing these issues because her body was not yet accustomed to the medication and that the symptoms would calm down. Victoria was still experiencing migraines. He prescribed an additional medication.

At this point, her mother was furious and even more concerned about Victoria's condition. Her daughter did not experience any illness growing up other than the typical childhood chicken pox and very rarely, a cold. She had perfect attendance eight of her twelve years of school and the absences for the four years she did not have perfect attendance were due to educational trips with her family.

Her mother, on her own, began reviewing Victoria's diet and realized an alarming discovery. Victoria had a part-time job at a local convenience store making the shakes and frothy drinks. Victoria began consuming flavored iced coffees instead of consuming her usual amount of water. The drinks were loaded with caffeine, sugar and corn syrup, artificial colors and flavors. These products were not part of Victoria's standard, healthy diet of fruits, vegetables, and lean meats she was served at home. She drank only water and tea without sugar at home. Additionally, she was eating processed foods at the school cafeteria and from the convenience store where she worked.

Her mother met with the professors to see how Victoria could complete the semester, considering her illness, if they could correct the situation by removing her from college for two weeks. Because Victoria had a 4.0 the first semester, three of the five professors agreed to work with Victoria upon her return to help her catch up. She had to withdraw from two classes.

Her mother took her home, returned her food consumption to fruits, vegetables, tea, and water. She did not purchase the second prescription and took Victoria off the anti-seizure medication by cutting the dose in half for the first three days, then by a third the next three days, down to a fourth the next three days, to an eighth the next two days, and no more medication after that.

Victoria returned to college after sixteen days at home. She had no more migraines and was not experiencing any side effects from the medication or being off the medication. Victoria's migraines were accidental self-inflicted dehydration—too many toxins and not enough nutrition.

Until I heard this account, I was unaware of how prominent migraine headache issues are for college students.

Dehydration is a major cause of headaches and migraines and can create serious health issues. Headaches are a symptom that the body is not getting the water and nutrients it needs to function properly. Persons consuming a healthy diet of fresh fruits and vegetables and appropriate alkaline water rarely experience headaches.

Reaction to a Food Additive or Medication

A variety of food additives, such as refined white sugar, aspartame, BHA, BHT, monosodium glutamate, artificial colors, and autolyzed yeast extract, for example, can cause a headache. The side effect of some prescription medications and hormone therapies are an additional cause of headaches and migraines.

These products are all toxic substances the body is struggling to combat. Therefore, they are excreted through urination, placing a higher demand on kidney function and resulting in dehydration.

Overconsumption of caffeine narrows the blood vessels and restricts blood flow. Theoretically, imagine if your blood vessels are the size of a drinking straw. Amazing amounts of fluid can flow through this straw. After consuming caffeine, imagine the blood vessels become the size of a stirrer straw. Using this illustration, you can imagine how much less blood can flow through the stirrer straw versus the drinking straw. Consuming high quantities of caffeine restricts the blood flow, even to the brain. When caffeine is eliminated, the blood vessels try to return to their normal size and blood flow is increased. This process creates a caffeine withdrawal headache or migraine.

Migraines and severe headaches from caffeine withdrawal are seemingly very well known. Caffeine users even announce their oncoming headache, "I'm getting a really bad caffeine withdrawal headache. I need some coffee now!" For others, they need soda to reduce headaches associated with caffeine and sugar addiction.

Nicotine, illegal drugs, alcohol, and other toxic substances create addiction, and withdrawal creates headaches and migraines.

In all of my years of research, I have never located information or heard any complaints about fruit or vegetable withdrawal headaches.

Headaches and migraines are very serious painful subjects. That being said, unless the headache or migraine is caused by a physical injury, nearly all others are self-inflicted due to chemical consumption or dehydration.

You may want to consider reviewing your diet and water intake before committing to a prescription medication for migraines that may cause more serious, permanent side effects.

Head or Neck Injury

Severe headache and migraines can also be associated with head or neck injuries. This contributing factor encompasses many injuries including concussions and whiplash.

Recovery from brain injuries may take weeks or even months. Rest and adequate nutrition assists with the recovery. However, headaches and migraines usually accompany these types of injuries due to swelling, pressure, and/or bleeding in the brain. Headaches from head injuries are common and appropriate due to the cause of the headache. *Extreme headaches or migraines, for any reason, and especially after head injuries, are cause for immediate medical attention.*

Neck injuries can often occur at the same time as the head injury. Many times, the stiffness associated with neck injuries subsides, but the headaches remain. A neck injury may not always be apparent on an X-ray because the spine is still aligned. However, the tissues, ligaments, tendons, nerves, and blood vessels may be impaired, causing headaches due to compromised functionality.

Consulting a chiropractor may be the best approach when no apparent medical explanation is attained. Chiropractic services can realign the spinal cord and help correct situations interfering with the autonomic nervous system that can cause a wide variety of physical and mental ailments due to restricted blood flow.

In some instances, headaches may not occur for a month or more after a low-speed impact such as a fender bender, a slip or fall that seems inconsequential, a rough ride on an all-terrain vehicle or a bicycle accident. While these events may seem insignificant at the time, when headaches occur on a daily basis several weeks later, the event may have caused a negative impact on the nervous system that will result in impaired blood flow. Also, muscle tension from these small incidents can cause headaches. Massage and chiropractic manipulation can provide relief for these situations.

21

Choose Wisely—Foods to Avoid

Making the decision to change your eating habits is a great first step. Deciding what food choices will help your health instead of harming it is the next decision. With all the confusing data surrounding you, those decisions can be overwhelming. This chapter is designed to help you make better choices by outlining what you need in your diet, what purchases you should avoid, and how your decisions will ultimately save you time, money, help reverse declining health, and maintain good health.

What *Not* to Eat...

1. Processed Meats. The chemicals used in processing, the sodium nitrites used as a preservative, and high-temperature rates for their preparation prompts additional dangers to these cancer-causing food items. *These processed products are now listed by the World Health Organization in the same cancer-causing category as cigarettes, alcohol, asbestos, arsenic, and plutonium.*[1] Processed meats are just not tasty enough to warrant intestinal cancer and severe heart disease.

- Bacon
- Hot Dogs
- Sausage
- Salami

2. Margarine is made from hydrogenated vegetable oils, artificial colors and flavors and deodorizers.

3. Meats with ractopamine (used to turn fat into lean protein as the animal matures). *Ractopamine is banned in 160 countries.* It is still used in the United States. Ractopamine is used in approximately 45 percent of pigs, 30 percent of cattle, and an unknown percentage in turkey. Since US meats containing ractopamine are not exported to 160 countries currently because the substance is banned due to the health issues it causes (it is estimated that approximately 20 percent of the ractopamine remains in the meat after the animal is slaughtered), US citizens are willing, able, and unknowing subjects to consume it every day and pay hard-earned money for it. Avoid non-organic beef, pork, and turkey products.

4. Soy products are *not* healthy for you. According to a report from the US Department of Agriculture, 94 percent of soy is genetically modified (GMO). In other cultures, only fermented soy products are used. In the United States, the products being marketed are unfermented; and due to the natural estrogen content in soy, can disrupt reproductive systems, causing multiple cancers, and various other disease symptoms.

Avoid all of these products:

- Soy milk, soy cheese, soy ice cream, soy yogurt
- Meatless products made of soy
- Soy protein
- Tofu
- Edamame
- Soy infant formula: "Soy infant formula puts your baby's health at risk. Nearly 20 percent of US infants are now fed soy formula, but the estrogens in soy can irreversibly harm your baby's sexual development and reproductive health. Infants fed soy formula take in an estimated five birth control pills' worth of estrogen every day. Infants fed soy formula have up to 20,000 times the amount of estrogen in circulation as those fed other formulas!"[2]
- Soy lecithin, in nearly everything from candy, condiments, soups, baked goods, imitation diary, imitation meats, protein powders, nutritional supplements, to name a few

- Mono-Diglycerides
- Soy, in some form, is in almost every processed product on the US market.

5. Shark, king mackerel, and swordfish contain the highest levels of mercury in fish. Mercury contributes to arthritis conditions.

6. Artificial sweeteners are artificial and some are neuro-toxins.

7. Soda and energy drinks are filled with synthetics and sugars and promote diabetes.

8. Refined white sugar is a chemically altered toxic version of real cane sugar.

9. Farm-raised fish and seafood are fed an unnatural diet of grains that makes their meat an unsightly grey color. In order to make it appetizing to you, the color is chemically altered so you will buy it. Farm-raised seafood is very dangerous and does not supply the vitamins and minerals of wild-caught fish and seafood. Farmed-raised salmon is the most dangerous.

10. Fast Food. AVOID; there are *no* safe, fast foods.

11. Non-organic corn is a genetically modified organism that is foreign to your body.

12. Non-organic tomatoes, tomato-based sauces of any kind; the skin of the tomato is removed with chemicals during processing.

13. Canned food contains little to no nutritional value.

14. Processed cheese is basically all chemicals.

15. ANYTHING microwaved; microwaving irradiates all forms of nutrition and changes the remaining foodstuffs into carcinogens.

The list of what to avoid is unbelievable. So what is there left to eat? Never fear, there are all sorts of wonderful, wholesome, nutritious foods!

What to Eat…

1. Raw, fresh organic fruits:

- Berries: blackberry, blueberry, cranberry, gooseberry, grapes, mulberry, strawberry, raspberry, tomato
- Tree Fruits: apple, apricot, cherry, peach, pear, plum, quince
- Citrus Fruits: banana, grapefruit, kiwi, lemon, lime, mango, orange, pineapple, tangerine
- Melons: cantaloupe, honeydew, watermelon

2. Raw, fresh organic vegetables:

- Broccoli
- Cabbage
- Carrot
- Cauliflower
- Celery
- Cress
- Cucumbers
- Kale
- Kohlrabi
- Leek
- Lettuce
- Mushrooms
- Onions
- Peppers
- Radish
- Spinach
- Watercress

3. Organic vegetables to prepare:

- Artichoke
- Asparagus
- Beets

- Brussel sprouts
- Collards
- Corn
- Gourds
- Okra
- Parsnip
- Rhubarb
- Rutabaga
- Shallots
- Squash
- Turnips
- Yams

4. Organic Dried Fruits

5. Organic Raw Nuts

6. Organic Dairy (in moderation)

- Butter
- Cheese
- Cottage Cheese
- Cream Cheese
- Half & Half
- Milk
- Yogurt, Plain

7. Organic Flour

- Buckwheat flour
- Cornmeal
- Flax meal
- Oat flour
- Rice flour
- Wheat flour
- Millet flour

- Spelt flour
- Barley flour
- Rye Flour

8. Organic Meats

- Beef
- Chicken
- Turkey
- Lamb

9. Wild-Caught Fish and Seafood

- Salmon
- Haddock
- Freshwater Trout
- Catfish
- Herring
- Sardines
- Scallops
- Shrimp
- Crab

10. Organic Pickles

11. Organic Olives

12. Organic Apple Cider Vinegar

13. Organic Olive Oil, Coconut Oil, Safflower Oil

14. Organic Coffee

15. Organic Loose Leaf Tea

16. Organic Herbs and Spices

17. Organic Eggs

18. Organic Lentils, Garbanzo Beans, Black Beans, White Navy Beans

19. Organic Agave Nectar

20. Organic Honey

21. Organic Tahini

Using organic ingredients, you can make your own: ice cream from frozen bananas, zucchini bread without yeast, tortillas, quesadillas, stir fry, baked chicken, omelets, smoothies, coffee creamer using organic half and half with organic flavors, yeast-free pizza crust, and so much more!

Dying an early death from ingesting artificial food is just the beginning. The long-term effects of consuming synthetic foods will be your legacy forever. Future generations will bear the ill-health affects from gene mutations caused by the "chemical cocktail" their parents, grandparents, and great-grandparents consumed in their lifetimes. You can already witness the apparent health effects of a chemical-laced, contaminated food supply by the increasing numbers of diseases and the number of friends and family you have known with the debilitating effects of cancer, diabetes, and heart disease. Disease is not inherited. But mutated genes will produce serious physical and psychological issues for future generations and the human race.

Fresh Fruit and Vegetable Diet Dangers for Some Individuals

While a fresh fruit and vegetable diet is the healthiest diet for humans, some people have current health issues that require attention prior to beginning this regimen.

People taking blood thinners: When taking blood thinners, the prescription dosage is based on your current diet. Choosing to consume more fresh vegetables than you are currently may affect the dosage. Vitamin K helps the blood to clot and inhibit excessive bleeding. Eating fresh fruits and vegetables provides nutrition and antioxidants, but knowing the facts and communicating with your health care professional can help you reach a balance that is right for you.

Severe diabetics. Ninety-five percent of all diabetes is directly correlated to the foods being consumed. When synthetic foods, sugars, and manmade carbohydrates are eliminated or significantly reduced, and food combining principles are followed, diabetes is no longer a health condition. For those individuals with severe alcoholism, gallstones, bacterial infections affecting the pancreas, a physical injury to the pancreas, and some autoimmune conditions contributing to diabetes, establishing a new diet high in fresh fruit and vegetables requires coordination with a health care professional. The body may not be able to effectively produce enough insulin for glucose metabolism.

Advanced disease disrupting bodily function. A fresh fruit and vegetable diet, once acute disease has eliminated the natural function of the kidneys and/or intestines, can only be consumed through juicing if permitted by your health care professional.

Metabolic disorders. People with genetic metabolic disorders responsible for dysfunctional or missing enzymes that disallow normal processing of sugars, certain vitamins and minerals, fats or proteins may not be candidates for a fresh fruit and vegetable diet. Consult your health care professional before attempting a diet change.

Other severe disease or inherited disorders. Your better health is the focus of this book. Rare forms of disease, allergies, and limitations of your body may preclude you from certain fruits or vegetables. Consult your health care provider or a natural health care professional if you have concerns or questions before proceeding with a fresh fruit and vegetable diet.

22

Organic Loose Leaf Tea Benefits

Green tea is the most studied plant on earth. And there are thousands of university studies to prove why it is so important. Green tea contains antioxidants proven to fight and even prevent certain types of cancer.

Let's keep this one thing in mind—not all green tea falls into this category. If the green tea you are ingesting is bottled, chilled, and sold by a local convenience store, it does not contain all the healthy properties. Most bottled green tea contains high fructose corn syrup, artificial flavors and colors. That is *not* green tea. Green tea contains EGCG (Epigallocatechin gallate) a type of cathechin. In its whole, organic, loose leaf form, green tea is a powerhouse for helping stop disease in its tracks.

The following is an abstract, the cover page, for a study on green tea.

> *An expanding body of preclinical evidence suggests EGCG, the major catechin found in green tea (Camellia sinensis), has the potential to impact a variety of human diseases. Apparently, EGCG functions as a powerful antioxidant, preventing oxidative damage in healthy cells, but also as an antiangiogenic and antitumor agent and as a modulator of tumor cell response to chemotherapy. Much of the cancer chemopreventive properties of green tea are mediated by EGCG that induces apoptosis and promotes cell growth arrest by altering the expression of cell cycle regulatory proteins, activating killer caspases, and suppressing oncogenic transcription factors and*

> *pluripotency maintain factors. In vitro studies have demonstrated that EGCG blocks carcinogenesis by affecting a wide array of signal transduction pathways including JAK/STAT, MAPK, PI3K/AKT, Wnt and Notch. EGCG stimulates telomere fragmentation through inhibiting telomerase activity. Various clinical studies have revealed that treatment by EGCG inhibits tumor incidence and multiplicity in different organ sites such as liver, stomach, skin, lung, mammary gland and colon. Recent work demonstrated that EGCG reduced DNMTs, proteases, and DHFR activities, which would affect transcription of TSGs and protein synthesis.* ***EGCG has great potential in cancer prevention because of its safety, low cost and bioavailability. In this review, we discuss its cancer preventive properties and its mechanism of action at numerous points regulating cancer cell growth, survival, angiogenesis and metastasis. Therefore, non-toxic natural agent could be useful either alone or in combination with conventional therapeutics for the prevention of tumor progression and/or treatment of human malignancies***.[1]
>
> http://www.ncbi.nlm.nih.gov/pubmed/21827739

The last section of this research abstract statement is printed in bold lettering because it contains the most compelling words you should have ever read about the benefits of green tea consumption. In other words, it states that green tea could be useful for the prevention of tumors and treatment of disease.

Organic Green Tea—the Secret Weapon against many diseases.

Organic green tea is the secret weapon against many diseases. It is so incredibly easy to enjoy healthy, real, organic green tea. Make it at home (three to four minutes from start to finish), add a frozen organic strawberry, raspberry, or fresh slice of orange if your palate has been conditioned to want a sweeter tea. You will enjoy all the benefits this incredible plant has to offer your better health.

Green tea helps level blood sugar, eradicates disease, provides antioxidants, provides a caffeine boost, and helps protect your heart and lower bad cholesterol levels. The EGCGs in green tea, helps protect cells from free radicals (substances foreign to the human body) and fortify healthy cells. *It is one of the most beneficial plants you can ingest.*

Many people in the United States are under the false impression that tea causes kidney stones. If that was the truth, how would any person in Asia or other parts of the world ever get out of bed? Kidney stones are painful and debilitating! Yet every day in Asia and other parts of the world, people drink four to five cups of organic green tea with no ill health effects—only positive ones. Real organic loose leaf tea does not cause kidney stones.

Red rooibos, an herb from South Africa, is a tea with abundant qualities. It does not originate from the same plant as green tea. Red rooibos (pronounced Roy-bus) contains fifty times more active antioxidants than green tea, but does not contain EGCGs. It is naturally caffeine-free, contains iron, calcium, potassium, copper, fluoride, manganese, zinc, magnesium, and alpha-hydroxy for your skin. It contains the highest levels of anti-aging properties of any plant on earth. Just imagine how much healthier you will be when you are consuming green tea and red rooibos tea! Of course, you can steep them together to get the benefits of both plants in the same cup of tea.

Black, oolong, and pu'erh tea may be considered inferior to green tea, but still pack an antioxidant punch worth buying. The phytochemicals of black tea contain benefits to protect your heart, DNA, teeth and bones, and antioxidants. It contains caffeine vital to prostate health and protects blood vessels. As a side note, it also helps with halitosis—bad breath. Just for the record, black tea does not cause kidney stones either.

White tea, the early leaves of green tea, *contains twenty times more antioxidants than green tea and contains all the benefits of green tea.* Because the leaves have not been fully exposed to the elements of weather conditions, white tea is lighter in taste.

While it may look lighter in the cup, it packs powerful amounts of antioxidants and EGCGs.

Herbal Teas

What about herbal teas? Let me explain the difference. Tea comes from certain plants: black, oolong, pu'erh, green, white, and yellow teas all come for the same plant, Camellia sinesis Herbal tea is marketed in two classes: herbal tea and herbal tea blends.

Herbal tea blends are a combination of herbs and tea leaves. Herbal tea does not contain any tea leaves. For example: green mint herbal blend tea is a combination of herbs (peppermint) and tea leaves (green tea). Peppermint herbal tea is comprised of just herbal leaves (peppermint). Tea leaves are combined with herbal roots, barks, or leaves to make a tea serve a particular purpose. For example: black teas, ginkgo, eyebright, and bilberry were combined in World War II and served as a tea for pilots to help fortify eyesight.

Herbal combinations are still written as medicinal prescriptions in many countries around the world. We are so progressive in the United States that our health is diagnosed by a symptom and a correlating pricy, toxic, pharmaceutical drug with disastrous side effects is prescribed instead of a low-cost, highly researched herb and corrective diet.

Drink organic loose leaf tea every day! Cup upon cup of it! Get your health back. Rebuke sugar. Rebuke processed foods. Rebuke high-priced, sugar and chemical-laced coffees. Drink real, organic leaves full of goodness and reap the benefits.

When purchasing herbs for their beneficial use, always choose certified organic dried herbs. They are in their purest form, without synthetic components, and have not been irradiated. Irradiation can destroy the medicinal compounds. If you are using these herbs for their medicinal benefit rather than just the taste, add them to food after it has been prepared because some of their effectiveness can be lost during the cooking or baking process.

At this point, we've learned:

1. The cells in the human body are preprogrammed to fight to stay alive.
2. The human body can repair itself.
3. Humans require nutrition for great health.
4. All disease is caused by the same thing—too many toxins, not enough nutrition.
5. Prescription medications only treat symptoms, not the problem.
6. Americans are overfed, undernourished, and diseased.
7. Our food supply is laden with dangerous chemicals.
8. What products to avoid that are proven to cause major health issues.
9. The products that are safe to consume.

The next chapters will help you understand what your body needs to expel the toxins and parasites in your body from years of eating synthetic and contaminated foods, and how to achieve and maintain better health for a lifetime.

23

Cleaning Up and Cleaning Out

When people move, they discard a variety of possessions. Old pots and pans, clothing that is never worn, expired foods, extras of every kind. Once accustomed to the new living area, the stock piles of useless materials once again accumulate in the new location. Moving into a new location forces us to deal with the hoarding situation in our living space. But today, let's address purging those useless or unused items because they have a negative effect on our health.

Cleaning up our eating habits is the first step to regaining health. Here is what that entails:

1. Cleaning out your refrigerator and freezer. If it is not a USDA Certified Organic product, throw it away. You can give it away if it makes you feel better. Please consider that you may be giving away carcinogenic products. To whom exactly does one give those?
2. Take a picture of your chemical collection before you begin the purging process.
3. Here is what nearly every person realizes when they clean out their refrigerator—the majority of the items they are tossing out were expired anyway!
4. You did not use them to begin with, so you do not have to spend the money replacing them.
5. Read some of the labels on those items as they are going into the trash bin. You will not feel so badly about throwing them away.

6. After the refrigerator is emptied, please take the time and wash it out. Clean the shelves, the bins, and the doors.
7. Now take another picture. Congratulations! Your new, healthy life just began.
   One excited woman who cleaned out her cupboards after attending one of our better health classes called to say she found an envelope with $500 in it from a Christmas gift she forgot she received eight years previously! She also found the old spice set she was gifted at her wedding. She had been married for twenty-two years and none of it had been opened. Her cabinets were filled with expired, non-usable items.
8. Repeat these same steps for the freezer, medicine cabinet, and laundry room.
9. Now clean out all the trash in your house, basement, and garage. Not only are you ingesting chemicals, you are breathing them. Piles of stuff collect dust particles from air fresheners, pets, make up, hair spray, deodorants, cleaning supplies, fossil fuels, perfumes and cologne, and dust from outside can leave unhealthy residue. Invite some friends to help you and make it a fun experience.
10. Donate the items you have not used and will never use to a nonprofit organization. The receipt will be tax deductible. Or have a yard sale. This may sound like a lot of work, but it is worth it to begin your new healthy life. If cleaning out the space you call home is that much work to do, your lifestyle is very unhealthy. Part of great health is emotional balance. Clearing out things that remind you of your old bad habits resets your outlook to accepting a new and healthier life.

Embark on a healthier lifestyle today. Make it fun. You may even laugh out loud when you realize that you have been housing condiments that expired two years ago!

Better health begins with you. Your body and your health are your most valuable assets.

24

Parasites

Now that you have cleaned up and cleaned out your living space, it is time to clean out your body. In this chapter, you will learn the health dangers of parasites associated with contaminated foods and water and how to rid your body of these dangerous organisms.

In 1993, Hulda Regehr Clark, PhD, ND, published *The Cure for All Cancers.* Along with chemicals and toxins being addressed in her book, she also explains the debilitating effects of parasites. An American television show premiered in 2009 called, "Monsters Inside Me." It was a documentary series recreating stories of ailments associated with parasites and other harmful toxins.

For many years, natural health professionals have addressed the growing health issues associated with parasitic occupation inside the human body. Parasite cleanses have been utilized to restore health even in the very worst cases of disease.

Consuming under cooked meats, eating raw fish, contaminated fruits and vegetables, and even consuming basic drinking water contribute to accumulating parasites in your body. Consuming commercial meats and fish products produces parasites in the intestines and liver. This parasitic activity creates somewhat of a blind spot for medical professionals. Unless the correct blood test is ordered to rule out parasites, assuming they know in advance which parasites to test for, some of these little critters can survive basic antibiotic treatment.

In 2014, CBS News released an article entitled, "CDC warns of common parasites plaguing millions in U.S." The article stated that in a report from the CDC, parasitic infection can lead to serious health issues and that parasites exist in the United States — not just in developing countries.[1]

Antibiotics are used for a wide range of parasitic infections and are often effective. Antibiotics do not eradicate all types of parasites; but there is, however, a natural way to rid the body of these incredulous monsters if you prefer not to use antibiotics and this way you can be certain that all of them are gone! By cleaning up your diet, you limit the possibility of re-infestation.

Parasite Cleanse

A valid parasite cleanse is done in steps so that each herb can produce the needed effects and is in a dose strong enough to accomplish destroying parasites without damaging the intestines or liver. Days upon days of diarrhea is a fecal cleanse, not a parasite cleanse. A fecal cleanse helps rid the body of excess toxic matter in the intestines in order to produce better nutrient absorption.

In order to kill parasites and rid them from your body, herbs are used that address each type of parasite. A very strong herbal combination of black walnut hull, cloves, and wormwood help destroy the pancreatic fluke, sheep liver fluke, human liver fluke, taenia solium, tapeworm, toxoplasma gondii, hookworm, maggots, entamoeba histolylica, and roundworm. These parasites reside in one organ or the other. The liver and/or intestines are both vulnerable. For five days, this strong mixture is designed to kill the parasites quickly and is taken twice a day.

Once the parasites are destroyed, drinking olive oil helps lubricate the bile ducts in the liver for ease of removing the parasitic debris. Herbs and tea help flush the dead parasites, larva, and eggs from the liver and fortify the liver tissue at the same time.

You may feel some discomfort as the parasites are flushing from the liver if they are larger in size or quantity. It is as if microscopic surgery is being performed as the body is naturally trying to expel the unwanted creatures.

You will be able to visibly identify the parasites in your excrement. Parasites range from small white worms, small see-through brown grape-like objects, small white balls that resemble tapioca pearls, to larger, flat, flukes in a variety of colors ranging from iridescent to white, brown, yellow, and red.

For those already suffering complications from parasites, including brain cysts and impaired vision, this cleanse may be combined with antibiotics.

Herbs such as bentonite clay, wheatgrass, barley grass, and spirulina address blood parasites, such as giardia, babesia, and flatworm blood fluke. Bentonite clay acts as a tiny sponge absorbing toxins in the liver and the blood. Wheatgrass and barley grass help purify the blood. Spirulina, considered a superfood, contains high amounts of vitamins and minerals, protein and is an alkaline substance that helps restore blood cells.

Parasites are silent, often misdiagnosed, killers. Unless you are maintaining a 7.4 pH balance in your body, you are serving as a human hotel for parasites.

Maintaining a cleaned up, cleaned out body is the next order of business. By eliminating farm-raised fish and seafood, non-organic meats and all fast foods, you can drastically limit your amount of parasitic exposure. People consuming large quantities of pork products, beef, and sushi report having eliminated the most parasites.

I spoke to a manager of the meat and seafood department at a well-known grocery chain. I was inquiring why I could not find wild-caught salmon at the store. The manager said that when the fish, and some meats, come into the back of the store, they put it in a heavy solution of salt in thirty or fifty-gallon plastic tubs resembling trash cans. The worms and parasites from the fish and meat rise to the surface of the tub and the employees scoop the worms and other debris off the top of the water and discard it. Then the water is emptied and the process is repeated.

If the quantity of worms and debris is still significant after the second time in the salt water, it is repeated until there is a comfort level that the fish or meat is acceptable for purchase. None of the additional sodium content for these products is reported on the label to the consumer. The manager said he became a strict organic vegetarian since the second day he was on the job.

I share this story because I was not aware these unwanted occupants in fish and meat existed when they arrive at their destination.

Fast Facts about Parasites

Parasitic infections affect millions of people in the United States every year.

- More than 300,000 people are infected with Trypanosoma cruzi, the cause of Chagas disease.
- At least 1,000 people are hospitalized with neurocysticercosis every year.
- Each year at least 70 people, most of them children, are blinded by the parasite that causes toxocariasis.
- More than 60 million persons are chronically infected with Toxoplasma gondii.
- Each year 1.1 million people are newly infected with trichomonas.[2]

Toxoplasma gondii is one of the most prevalent parasitic infections in the United States. It is introduced into the body by consuming undercooked, contaminated meat, or accidentally ingesting it due to contaminated kitchen appliances, utensils, or unwashed hands after touching the contaminated source.

Cat feces attributes to this parasitic infection through improper handwashing or personal sanitation after cleaning the feline's litter box. Pregnant women are warned to wear gloves when emptying and cleaning a litter box. Owning a cat does not conclude that you will have this parasite.

Eating after gardening without properly washing your hands or consuming fruits and vegetables without washing them first can contribute to parasite ingestion through contaminated soil.

Indications of infection can include muscle aches and swollen glands resembling flu-like symptoms. Severe cases of infection can cause serious damage to the brain and eyes. Other organs can be affected as well.

Toxocariasis exists in the feces of cats and dogs, predominately. The larvae of the roundworm can occupy a human when there is direct contact with the infected feces and accidental ingestion happens when proper hand cleansing does not occur. Ingesting infected undercooked meats, such as rabbit, sheep, or chicken, can also deliver this parasite. Contaminated soil in pet parks and playgrounds pose an additional risk of exposure to this parasite, especially for children.

Untreated toxocariasis creates multiple health hazards including respiratory issues, headaches, insomnia, loss of appetite, and in severe causes, blindness and seizures. Because the symptoms of this infection are so varied, diagnosis of toxocariasis can be difficult.

Neurocysticercosis is a result of an infestation of the larval cystic form of a pork tapeworm. It is attributed as a major cause of acquired seizures and epilepsy. With at least one thousand people being hospitalized annually in the United States with neurocysticercosis, it is not classified as a wide-spread parasitic infection and can be treated effectively when properly diagnosed.

Chagas disease is caused by a parasite, Trypanosoma cruzi. The parasite leaves infected feces behind after biting the person. The bite does not cause the disease; the feces entering the body through the eyes, nose, mouth, or the bite area is what precipitates infection. Other ways of attaining Chagas disease is through contaminated foods, organ transplant, blood transfusion, or from a mother to her newborn.

Symptoms include flu-like symptoms, including fever, rash, or swollen eyelid. These parasites prefer to bite the face near the eyes or mouth. Parasitic activity can wreak havoc on your body and sometimes, those devilish little things, are difficult to diagnosis. Heavy meat eaters and persons consuming diets heavy in sushi experience unexplained ailments that I attribute to parasites.

Trichomonas is a sexually transmitted parasite that can be treated effectively with antibiotics.

Parasite Exposure when Traveling

Traveling to developing countries evokes a concern about parasites for many people and is a legitimate concern. Before your international adventure begins, doing some research to understand the parasitic dangers is highly recommended.

For example, Punta Cana in Dominican Republic is considered a paradise vacation. Yet, tourists are warned of the dangers of dengue fever, malaria, and traveler's diarrhea.[3] Visitors are instructed not to consume the water or even brush their teeth with it.

When traveling to developing countries, use the following precautions to limit your exposure to parasites and other bacteria: Use bottled water to:

- wash your face and hands.
- brush your teeth.
- rinse your hands and face after taking a shower because local water can cause a variety of health issues. Do not consider your hands "clean" after showering.

Following these simple steps can help limit your exposure to water-related parasites.

The world is a beautiful playground. Parasites should not inhibit your traveling plans. With easy access to current information for any foreign destination, you can travel prepared with mosquito and other insect repellants. Choose adventures to areas with less probability of exposure and learn to use only bottled water for even the slightest occasion requiring water.

25

Seek Valid Natural Health Advice

Locating a valid practitioner can create a little bit of concern when you are beginning your natural health journey. Having a list of credentials associated with various accredited college and university degrees in natural health practices can help eliminate the stress of knowing who to trust for advice.

Degree and Credential Initials

Acupuncture Physician - AP
Doctor of Ayurvedic Medicine & Surgery - DAMS
Doctor of Chiropractic - DC
Doctor of Holistic Natural Health - PhD
Doctor of Naturopathic Medicine - NMD
Doctor of Naturopathy - ND
Doctor of Natural Health & Nutrition - PhD
Doctor of Oriental Medicine - OMD or DOM
Doctor of Physical Therapy - DTP

One of the most challenging obstacles in natural health is knowing who trust and what to believe. Locating a natural health care professional with a degree can help eliminate this frustration. Taking critical health advice from the guy down the street who never completed high school but cultivates a beautiful herb garden does not qualify as seeking advice from a health care professional. People can be opinionated and freely offer their advice about handling health issues. This advice may inadvertently create health issues.

This valuable advice from my adolescence has treated me very well over the years. I was advised to never take mortgage advice from someone who has never had one! Seeking advice for a mortgage requires speaking with a qualified financial professional. Likewise, never take remodeling advice from someone who has never held a wrench or a hammer! Understanding the requirements for replacement of your heating and air conditioning system necessitates the advice of a qualified professional.

Following a natural protocol for great health should not be reduced to following the instructions of a friend or coworker who has never studied the complexities or complications involved with eradicating disease or the complications that may surface from withdrawing from certain medications before the body is well enough to sustain a healthy existence.

I have witnessed people attempting to change their health for the better only to watch their health worsen because they relied solely on the information provided to them from someone selling an herbal product. They trusted the salesperson who had no health training, just training on how to sell the product and be rewarded for it. There is no one product that exists on this planet that is made into a pill or packet of powder that can restore your health. There are many salespeople trying to convince health seekers that there are. Miracle pills do not exist. They are not made in nature.

I called a vitamin company in 2016 to find out what plant source they used to create the vitamin E supplement I located in a pharmacy. I wanted to be sure that it did not contain soy. The customer service representative answering the phone could not answer my question and offered to have someone return my call with that information. Two weeks later I received the return call and was informed that the product was 100 percent synthetic and totally safe for me to use because soy was not an ingredient.

The words "safe" and "100 percent synthetic" do not belong in the same sentence! The woman returning the call thought I was inquiring about the soy content because it could possibly cause an allergic reaction.

Knowing the facts about a product and exactly what it is made of is critical for better health. It contradicts all your hard work to eliminate synthetic and processed foods only to start putting synthetic and processed products back into your diet because they are disguised as vitamins or beneficial herbal supplements.

The whole purpose of doing something different for your health is to treat the cause, not the symptom. Taking a supplement to treat a symptom puts you right back on the same track you were on with the medical community.

Treating the cause will always allow you to focus your time and money on being well. True health cannot come from a pill, even an herbal pill. Herbs in a raw, dried organic form can be consumed in foods or made into teas. They can provide a valuable addition to your natural health protocol. Herbal pills and capsules normally go through a heated process and are rarely made of whole foods.

True health comes with maintaining an alkaline/acid balance in your body. Teas and herbs can aid in removing toxins, boosting antioxidants and decreasing inflammation, but are not replacements for the consumption of fresh, raw organic fruits and vegetables, raw nuts and seeds. There is no one item or herbal remedy that can reverse all the damage caused by years of destructive eating habits. They must be incorporated with a constructive, balanced diet.

For your better health, learn to read ingredient labels on herbal and vitamin supplements. Let's review a Magnesium supplement, for example. The other ingredients listed on the label are:

Cellulose gel – made from wood pulp or cotton

Croscarmellose Sodium – made by soaking crude cellulose in sodium hydroxide (better known as lye) then interacting the cellulose with another substance based in chlorine

Stearic Acid – made from fatty acids from hydrogenated vegetable or animal oils

Hydroxypropyl Methylcellulose – made from lye treated cellulose, reacted with methyl chloride and propylene oxide (a flammable liquid)

Magnesium Stearate – is basically the same as stearic acid. This ingredient goes by multiple names.

Silicon Dioxide – known as silica

Color Added – what color and from what source we might ask! The label just states as an ingredient: color added.

Polyethylene Glycol – can be synthetic or made from vegetable or animal bases. Used as a laxative.

Triethyl Citrate – ester of citric acid, made from sucrose, derived mainly from corn

Polysorbate 80 – made from sorbitol (made from some fruits, corn or seaweed) and oleic acid (fatty acids from vegetable or animal fats)

After reading this list, perhaps you may want to get your magnesium from cacao, fruits, vegetables and nuts! This product contains some heavy duty synthetic components. And there is no way of knowing if the magnesium content is synthetic.

Many vitamin and mineral supplements contain a variety of synthetic and dangerous additives. In addition, the actual vitamin and mineral you require may be synthetically processed making the entirety of the supplement synthetic!

Many liquid vitamin and herbal supplements use synthetic preservatives, such as sodium benzoate, to prolong their shelf life. To eliminate the possibility of bacteria or spoilage, sodium benzoate destroys all active ingredients! So whatever the ultimate, amazing, cure-everything, healing substance was supposed to be, it cannot exist in the presence of sodium benzoate. If the product contains certain preservatives, you are being sold a product with no active, healthy ingredients and it can, in fact, cause damage to your health.

Save your money and buy some fresh organic fruits and vegetables instead of synthetic vitamins.

26

Testimonials

The following are testimonials I received over the years that attest to the information provided to you in this book. I offer them as proof that changing your eating habits and lifestyle is possible and encourage you to take steps to become a healthier you.

From Angela: My Life-and-Death Decisions

A year ago, I was diagnosed with breast cancer. It devastated me. They told me that if they removed both breasts I would never have to worry about it happening again. I just got engaged four weeks earlier and couldn't even consider that option.

I went to a specialist to get a second opinion. An older lady in the waiting room, Pam, told me about using organic products at Gardens by Grace and beating breast cancer. She could see how upset I was about making a life-or-death decision. At least, that is how I was looking at it.

The next day I went to Gardens by Grace. I started drinking the Big C Total Body Fortifier tea and eating more organic fresh fruits and vegetables. I rested more, drank more water, gave up all sodas, and never ate food from a box. When three months passed, my family starting getting furious because I wasn't doing anything to save myself from cancer. They wanted me to have the operation.

I went back to the specialist five months later for another test. They found NO SIGNS OF CANCER. I still have both healthy breasts, and the only scars are the emotional ones from being scared out of my mind that I was going to be mutilated and then die before I turned 35.

Thanks for doing what you do DK. You make a difference. You helped save my life.

From Janice: My Cancer Is Gone!

Dear Ms. Guyer:

I am not sure if you will remember me or not, but I just needed to say thank you for all you have done to help my health. I followed all the instructions you gave me, did the cleanse, started eating the list of fruits and veggies, drinking the Big C Total Body Fortifier Tea, and I just had my six-month follow-up appointment. MY CANCER IS GONE! Not reduced or shrunk, GONE!

I think about how awesome it is that I prayed I would find a way to get healthy and get rid of this terrifying cancer—and the next day my sister took me to the "soap" store. I found new hope and new life there. We joke that the "soap" store really cleaned me up!

Your products do what they are supposed to and I feel so blessed that you are here in this little town and I didn't have to drive hours to find help. Thank you again for everything and for helping me find a new healthy life and a stronger faith in God.

From Don: I Have My Life Back

I never thought my health could improve so much so fast just by using some herbs and teas and changing the way I eat. The cleanse was a challenge because I tend to procrastinate. But after making it through that, using the Big C Total Body Fortifier tea, my headaches are gone, my blood pressure is stable, I stopped taking pills to get to sleep at night, and I feel better and have more energy.

It is no wonder I had to stand in line for a chance to talk to you. I read the testimonials on the wall while I waited, hoping I could get some of the same wonderful results all those people were describing. I did! And I wanted you to know about it. I will be a customer for life!

Thank you for caring and taking the time to help me. I feel like I have my life back.

From David: Your Tea Blends

I have not written a testimonial for a product at any time in my life. Your Big C Total Body Fortifier Tea deserves one. Actually, it deserves a place in medical history books.

I purchased a pound of it to help with the effects of Lyme Disease. Using the Big C tea, I have energy, limited aches and pains, and an opportunity to care for myself instead of depending on others to care for me. I have used a variety of products advertised to help with Lyme Disease complications. This tea works.

Coming to your store and talking with such knowledgeable people has given hope and new life to me and my family. Thank you for a wonderful product.

From Tess: Fibromyalgia

I grew up with a mother who treated taking medicine like it was a status symbol—the more pills, the better. When I was diagnosed with fibromyalgia at age 28, my head was spinning and the idea of spending the rest of my life in my mother's medicinal shadow terrified me.

When my friend Marci told me about your store and her success using your products, I became determined to find a natural solution. How lucky am I? After doing the cleanse and using the Groovin' Again and Big C Total Body Fortifier teas, I have not had one bed-ridden day, no medicines, and I feel like I can take on the world. Thank you so much for dedicating your life to helping the "seekers" get healthy!

P.S. Please dedicate one of your newsletters to telling folks that they don't have to rely on medicines to heal and help their bodies. From the amount of people in your store, I am sure you have quite an extensive list to email. One by one, the news will spread that a natural approach can work and work very well, and it is much cheaper than medicine without the hidden side effects. I love your store.

From Marcus: If You Can Read, Read This!

When I came to Gardens by Grace for the first time, I was in severe pain and felt awful all the time. I heard the commercial on the radio about better health. So I asked DK what natural remedy might make me feel better. She asked if I had ever done a cleanse.

A cleanse? I was 368 pounds and I stand 6'3". I'm not a little guy. I power-lifted for eight years. A cleanse sounded absolutely stupid to me. She could read my reaction and went in detail explaining how, why, etc., and showed me pictures of parasites in a book. Then she asked the determining question, "How often do you eat at McDonald's?" Oops. She's not gonna be happy with my response. I said maybe twice a week, but the truth is, it was almost every day. I would eat four of the $1 double cheeseburgers for lunch with fries.

She whipped out a paper with instructions, zoomed through the store collecting the items and told me how to do the cleanse. She told me sternly that considering my stature and eating habits, I could experience some pain during this cleanse because the dead parasites had to come out of the liver. I huffed that I was used to pain, no problem. I was a big boy, right?

Two months later, I came back to see Ms. DK and talk to her about her cleanse. I thought I was having a heart attack I hurt so bad.* While I was in the emergency room, they made me use a bed pan because they were not sure the stability of my condition. The nurse screamed out loud when she observed a six inch parasite in my stool! She made me look at it and tell her what kind of joke I was playing! I told her I was doing a parasite cleanse and that it was supposed to kill parasites in the liver and such. After the X-rays and a bunch of doctors having no idea what was wrong with me, I checked myself out.

After actually seeing the parasite, I remembered what DK said about experiencing some pain. In a matter of one week (took off work using vacation for this), I passed 4 gall stones, 2 kidney stones, countless very large parasites, and I was only half way through the cleanse. I lost 22 pounds in the first 10 days of the cleanse and hadn't made it to the intestinal part of the cleanse yet.

To make a very long, more than disgusting testimonial a page long instead of a novel, I eliminated stuff from my body that would make a warrior faint. I could barely stomach the thought that I was a walking sewage plant. I have not been to a fast food establishment since the cleanse, and I will never go there again. I am supposed to be doing the cleanse again in September (DK said to do it again in 6 months) but I am not gonna do it until October when I have vacation—just in case.

I am now 262 pounds and full of energy. I do not have the pain, stopped taking ALL my medications for cholesterol, diabetes, sleep, migraines—and only use natural remedies and eat organic foods. If you want to feel better, do the cleanse. The pain you experience to get those terrible creatures out of your body is worth it. Kill those parasite bastards and get your healthy life back.

**Not everyone experiences severe pain going through the cleanse. In this case, Marcus consumed a heavy diet of low-quality fast food meats for every meal daily.*

From Sharon: Downward Spiral

I was on seven medications and the side effects were killing me. Literally. At night, I used to lay there and tried to scheme how I would crash my car on the way to or from work so no one would know I took my life. I was that desperate.

I went to the doctor because I felt tired all the time. My downward spiral started when I took the first medication for my thyroid. Then I got an irregular heartbeat and chest pains and started my second medication. The third was for fibromyalgia. Then I needed a sleeping pill because I was tired all the time but couldn't sleep. Then my mood swings and depression got out of hand so they prescribed another med. Then two more for high blood pressure and cholesterol. I felt miserable and was getting worse by the day instead of better.

A friend at work begged me to go to Gardens by Grace. She was getting scared for me and my declining health. The side effects of three of the medications I was taking included thoughts of suicide and hurting myself. The medications that were supposed to HELP me were causing me to lose my mind and seriously consider taking my own life.

DK's kindness and information led me on a path that turned out to be remarkable. I am not on any medications anymore! I have my life back. I did the cleanse and used the Big C Total Body Fortifier tea — she combined a special green and red tea combination just for me so I would like it — to help my immune system. But there is another part to this story.

I would put aside my whole first paycheck of the month ($485) plus $200 of my husband's paycheck just to pay for doctor bills, specialist appointments, and medication. After getting out of the medication rut, we have been able to save all that money because we just kept putting it aside in case the natural program didn't work. I will be medication-free for fifteen months on July 18. We have $10,285 in our "pill pot" savings account!

But there's more. The doctor's office hounded me two to three times a week to come in to get another prescription when it ran out. When I told them I wasn't taking it anymore they got mad! Furious! They did not care that I was feeling better. They had no interest that my feelings of suicide were gone. They just wanted their money.

Life is what you make it. If you want to feel better, then do something about it. Take the first step. Save your own life because there are people in your life who love you and need you.

From a Registered Nurse: Sick of being Sick

My health has been deteriorating over the past four-five years. I am a registered nurse. That's right. I work in the medical field where you think I would be surrounded by healthy people. That is not a reality. I know more nurses who are as sick or worse than our patients! Many of them are taking seven-eight prescriptions a day. My crazy younger sister would tell me to get off the medicines and use natural products and I would feel better. Well, I stayed stuck on my own ideas that I had the medical education and she knew nothing; she never went any further in education than high school.

During our family Thanksgiving gathering, I was miserable. Headaches, tired achy all over, pain in my abdomen, my face was breaking out, I would have diarrhea one day then constipation for four days, my legs would swell, I was moody, and the list goes on and on. I was scheduled for another CAT scan the following week to see what was causing me so much pain. I told my extended family that I was sick of being sick. My sister simply said, "I will help you. I am tired of seeing you this way."

That is how we ended up at Gardens by Grace on Black Friday. I gained so much knowledge that day. I did the cleanse, I stopped eating certain foods, I dropped 18 pounds, and I felt energetic enough to walk the Ice Fest route this past weekend. The people in your store were so friendly and truly, genuinely interested in helping me achieve better health, that going to work every day and pushing medicines has become difficult because I received a NEW education through my sister and your store! Natural products really DO work. Medicines make you sick. They only treat the symptoms, not the cause.

We stopped by during the Ice Fest event in town, and looking at the testimonials on the walls, I knew mine needed to be there also. Gardens by Grace has the right products, the right attitude, and the right information to help anyone get their health back on track. I love this store!

P.S. I didn't sign my name because I work at a hospital.

From Kiesha: You Literally Saved My Life

I owe you all a debt of gratitude I can never repay. For the past eight years, I suffered unexplained pain, restless nights, no energy, headaches, and basic depression because of my situation. When a coworker, Anne, recommended Gardens by Grace, I was reluctant and even a bit scared to try something new. My attitude was so low and I felt like the world had beaten me down so far I would never have a chance to experience life the way my friends and family were able to. I was always too tired and in too much discomfort to do the fun things they did in the evenings and weekends.

I just counted myself lucky that I could still go do my job. When Anne invited me to go to the store with her after work one day, I refused, believing that no one could help me. It would be a waste of time. But she was persistent enough to get me out the door. Once I was there, and in the midst of other customers saying how much they loved the products and how pleased they were with the results, my attitude began to change. Maybe there was some hope for me.

When I read the testimonial about the 34-year-old with cancer, I realized that I did have something to be thankful for (at least I didn't have that battle) and that my health was my responsibility. After describing my ailments and the prescriptions I was taking, a very nice lady explained that I couldn't fix everything overnight and that, just as medicine takes awhile to work, so would a natural remedy. The difference was the side effects of the medications would diminish and as I began the natural journey, my overall situation would improve.

Well, that was an understatement of huge proportion! After only three weeks drinking some tea and adding some spices to my food, my headaches started to go away. Then I started sleeping at night without taking any pills! My mood swings calmed down, my energy started increasing, and people keep asking me what I did differently because I started looking better!

To make this really long story short, I will be a lifelong customer and forever indebted to you and my friend, Anne. I went from taking eleven prescription drugs to zero in six months. I even made plans to go to the beach with some friends next weekend. Please, please, please post this testimonial somewhere in hopes that if people like me need help moving forward and taking responsibility for their own health, they might read this and not be so hesitant. You all are wonderful. Thank you again. You literally saved my life!

27

Final Thoughts

When you comprehend the fact that you are an expendable guinea pig being manipulated into a life of disease by pharmaceutical and chemical companies, it should illicit grave concern for your life, the lives of your family, and future generations. While large corporations gain wealth and power, your healthy choices are limited by their greed. Changing your habits and demanding uncontaminated choices gives you a voice, and ultimately, a chance to alter the current status quo for food choices in the United States to become better.

We live as synthetic children parented by the masters of marketing. When we act as if we have no dedication to our own preservation as a healthy society, we create the opportunity for any corporation to manipulate our declining health into a profitable venture.

I hope you will choose to remedy your diet to reflect a positive change, share the truth about real health with someone else, and live a healthy and wonderful life.

28

Food Ingredients' List

This comprehensive ingredients list, created by Wanda Embar, is included as a helpful resource. It contains information about the substances utilized to create ingredients used in the foods we eat.

Please note that:

- Some substances in this list (even those marked as vegan) might have been tested on animals.
- Some substances in this list (even those marked as vegan) can be undesirable for use because of associated health problems.
- Ingredients that companies define as "synthetic" can have animal ingredients as their starting raw material. One example is vitamin D3, which can be derived from animal ingredients like lanolin, even though the company has defined it as "synthetic."

(A) = Animal ingredient
(V) = Vegan ingredient (synthetic, vegetable, or plant/mineral-derived)
(B) = Ingredient exists in both animal and vegan versions

Acesulfame/Acesulfame Potassium/Acesulfame K/Ace K (V): an artificial sweetener. Also sold commercially as Sunette or Sweet One. It has no nutritional value or calories. Might increase cancer risk in humans.

Acetate (B): vitamin A

Actinidin (V): enzyme derived from kiwi fruit used in the food industry

Adrenaline (B): comes from the adrenal glands of hogs, cattle and sheep

Agar-agar (agar) (V): extracted from seaweeds

Albumen/Albumin (B): a group of simple proteins composed of nitrogen, carbon, hydrogen, oxygen, and sulfur that are soluble in water. Albumen is usually derived from egg whites (ovalbumin), but can also be found in plasma (serum albumin), milk (lactalbumin) and vegetables and fruits.

Allantoin (B): can be extracted from urea (the urine of most animals, including humans) or from herbs such as comfrey or uva ursi

Allura Red (B): FD&C Red 40

Aloe Vera (V): compound expressed from the leaf of the aloe plant

Alpha hydroxy acids (B): naturally-occurring chemicals derived from fruit or milk

Aluminum Hydroxide (V): manufactured by dissolving bauxite in sodium hydroxide

Aluminum Sulfate (V): used in the purification of drinking water and in the paper manufacturing industry. Produced by adding aluminum hydroxide to sulfuric acid.

Ambergris (A): morbid concretion obtained from the intestine of the sperm whale

Amino acids (B): "building blocks" of proteins

Amniotic fluid (A): fluid surrounding the fetus within the placenta

Amylase (B): enzyme derived from either animal (usually porcine pancreas), fungal, bacterial, or plant source (barley malt).

Anchovy (A): small fish of the herring family

Angora (A): fiber obtained from angora rabbits

Annatto (V): a vegetable dye from a tropical tree

Anthocyanins (V): water-soluble plant pigments

Arachidonic acid (A): liquid unsaturated fatty acid found in the liver, brain, glands, and fat of animals

Artificial (B): product made by humans from natural ingredients. Like synthetic products, it would not exist without human intervention.

Ascorbic Acid (V): a water-soluble vitamin found in vegetables and fruits or made synthetically

Aspartame (V): an artificial sweetener known as NutraSweet prepared from aspartic acid and phenylalanine (vegan according to the NutraSweet Company)

Aspartic Acid (B): Amino succinate acid. An amino acid occurring in animals and plants usually synthesized from glutamate for commercial purposes.

Aspic (A): savory jelly derived from meat and fish

Astrakhan (A): skin of stillborn or very young lambs from a breed originating in Astrakhan, Russia

Baker's Yeast (V): common name for yeast used as a leavening agent in bakery products

Bauxite (V): an aluminum ore, the main commercial source of aluminum

Bee pollen (A): microsporic grains in seed plants gathered by bees then collected from the legs of bees

Beeswax (B): wax usually obtained from melting honeycomb with boiling water, straining it, and cooling it. Can be manufactured synthetically.

Beet Sugar (V): sugar derived from sugar beets

Benzoic Acid (V): produced by the oxidation of toluene with an oxygen-containing gas in the presence of a heavy metal oxidation catalyst

Beta Carotene (V): the carotene that's important in the diet as a precursor of vitamin A. It is used as a food coloring. Note: some manufacturers use gelatin as a stabilizer for beta carotene to help it disperse in liquids. The gelatin won't necessarily be listed in the ingredient list of the product

Betatene (V): trade name for a naturally occurring blend of carotenes, including beta carotene. It is derived from the sea algae, Dunaliella salina.

Bone/Bonemeal (A): animal bone

Bone char(coal)/Boneblack (A): animal bone ash. Black residue from bones calcined in closed vessels. Used especially as a pigment or as a decolorizing absorbent in sugar manufacturing.

Bone phosphate (A): manufactured from animal bones

Bonito (A): smaller relative of the tuna fish. Used as an ingredient in Japanese cuisine. See katsuobushi.

Brawn (A): boiled meat, ears, and tongue of pig

Brewer's Yeast (V): live yeast used in beer brewing or deactivated yeast obtained as a by-product of beer brewing and used as a nutritional yeast product

Brilliant Blue FCF (B): FD&C Blue 1

Bristle (A): stiff animal hair, usually from pigs

Bromelain (V): enzyme derived from the fruit, stem, and leaves of the pineapple plant

Butane (V): gaseous component of natural gas; extracted during the production of petroleum products like gasoline or produced from crude oil

Calcium Carbonate (B): tasteless, odorless powder that occurs naturally in marble, limestone, coral, eggshells, pearls or oyster shells

Calcium Chloride (V): odorless white to off-white granules, powder or liquid. Produced in a variety of ways, including treating limestone with hydrochloric acid, combining limestone with a sodium chloride solution and by concentrating and purifying naturally occurring brines from salt lakes and salt deposits. Has many uses including additive for foods, deicing agent for sidewalks and roads, water treatment.

Calcium Disodium EDTA (V): a synthetic preservative used to prevent crystal formation and to retard color loss. Has caused health problems and is banned in Australia and certain other countries.

Calcium Hydroxide (V): also known as slaked lime. Used as acidity regulator in drinks and frozen foods or as a preservative. Produced commercially by treating lime with water or by mixing calcium chloride and sodium hydroxide.

Calcium Lactate (B): the calcium salt of Lactic Acid

Calcium Phosphate (B): (Monobasic, Dibasic and Tribasic) a mineral salt found in rocks and bones. Used as an anti-caking agent in cosmetics and food, mineral supplement, abrasive in toothpaste and jelling agent. Also known as calcium rock.

Calcium Stearate (B): mineral calcium with stearic acid

Calcium stearoyl-2-lactylate (B): the calcium salt of the stearic acid ester of lactyl lactate

Candelilla wax (V): a vegetable wax obtained from candelilla plants

Cane Sugar (B): sugar obtained from sugarcane. In some countries (like the US), cane sugar is often processed through boneblack.

Capiz (A): shell

Caramel (B): used as a coloring. Manufactured by heating carbohydrates with or without acids or alkalis. Possible carbohydrates used are corn, beet sugar, cane sugar, wheat, or potatoes. The great majority of caramel is derived from corn and will be vegan. However, some caramel is derived from cane sugar and not necessarily vegan.

Carbamide (B): Urea

Carbon Black (B): Vegetable Carbon

Carbonic Acid (V): weak acid formed when carbon dioxide combines with water

Carmine/Carminic acid (A): Cochineal

Carnauba wax (V): wax obtained from the leaves of the carnauba palm

Carotene (V): red-orange pigment found in plants and fruits, consisting of alpha carotene, beta carotene, and gamma-carotene. Can be produced synthetically, derived from carrots or sea algae.

Carrageenan (V): extracted from various red algae and especially Irish Moss

Casein (A): milk protein

Cashmere (A): fine wool from the cashmere goat and wild goat of Tibet

Castor/Castoreum (A): obtained from anal scent gland of the beaver

Castor oil (V): vegetable oil expressed from the castor bean

Catalase (B): enzyme that decomposes hydrogen peroxide into water and oxygen. Derived from cattle liver or fungus and used in the food industry.

Catgut (A): dried and twisted intestines of sheep or horse
Caviar(e) (A): roe of the sturgeon and other fish
Cellulose (V): principal component of the fiber of plants. Cellulose is usually obtained from wood pulp or cotton (which contains about 90% cellulose).
Cetyl alcohol (B): found in Spermaceti or synthetic
Cetyl palmitate (B): Spermaceti, can be synthetic
Chalk (B): Calcium Carbonate
Charcoal (B): charred bone or wood
Chitin (A): organic base of the hard parts of insects and crustacea, e.g., shrimps, crabs
Chamois (A): soft leather from the skin of the chamois antelope, sheep, goats, deer, etc.
Cholecalciferol (A): vitamin D3
Cholesterol (A): steroid alcohol occurring in all animal fats and oils, nervous tissue, egg yolk, and blood
Chondroitin (B): used in products designed to help alleviate the effects of osteoarthritis. Produced synthetically or derived from the cartilage of cows, pigs, sharks, fish or birds.
Chymosin (B): Rennin
Chymotrypsin (A): enzyme primarily derived from ox pancreas
Cinnamic Acid (V): obtained from cinnamon leaves, coca leaves, balsams like storax, or isolated from a wood-rotting fungus. Can be made synthetically.
Citric Acid (V): derived from citrus fruits; since the 1920s commercially produced by fermenting sugar solutions with the microorganism Aspergillus niger. Main raw materials used in the production are corn-derived sucrose and molasses.
Civet (B): substance painfully scraped from glands in the anal pouch of the civet cat
Coal tar (V): thick liquid or semisolid tar obtained from bituminous coal (= soft coal)
Cochineal (Carmine, Carminic acid, Natural Red 4)(A): red pigment extracted from the crushed carcasses of the female cochineal insect, a cactus-feeding scale insect
Cod liver oil (A): oil extracted from the liver of cod and related fish

ColFlo 67 (V): modified food starch derived from waxy maize. Used in frozen foods and canned products. Often labeled as "Food Starch – Modified"

Collagen (A): protein found in most connective tissues, including bone, cartilage, and skin. Usually derived from cows or chickens.

Collagen hydrolysate (A): purified protein derived from animal sources; produced by breaking down gelatin to smaller protein fragments

Colors/Dyes (B): Can be from plant, animal, and synthetic sources. Most FD&C and D&C colors are derived from coal tar. Coal tar in itself is considered a vegan product. However, coal tar derivatives cause frequent allergic reactions, like skin rashes and hives. Also shown to cause cancer in animals. For this reason, colors and dyes are continuously tested on animals. That's why FD&C and D&C colors and dyes can generally not be considered vegan and I mark them as (B).

Confectioner's Glaze (A): Resinous Glaze

Coral (A): hard calcareous substance consisting of the continuous skeleton secreted by coelenterate polyps for their support and habitation

Cornstarch/Corn starch (V): starch derived from dried corn kernels

Corn Syrup (V): form of glucose made from corn starch; used as a sweetener

Corticosteroid/Cortisone (B): steroid hormones secreted by the adrenal cortex and their synthetic analogs

Cottonseed oil (V): fixed oil derived from the seeds of the cultivated varieties of the cotton plant

Crospovidone (V): Polyvinylpyrrolidone

Curcumin (V): Colorant derived from turmeric

Cysteine, L-Form (B): amino acid that oxidizes to form cystine **(B):** amino acid found in the hair protein keratin

Dashi (fish broth) (A): stock made from fish and seaweed. Used in Japanese cuisine.

D&C Colors (B): colors certified safe for use in drugs and cosmetics, but not in food by the FDA (the US Food and Drug Administration). See Colors/Dyes.

Dextrin (V): prepared by heating dry starch or starch treated with acids. Can be produced from the starch of corn, potatoes, or rice.

DiCalcium Phosphate (B): (Dibasic calcium phosphate, Dicalcium orthophosphate) Dibasic form of calcium phosphate

Dihydroxyacetone (B): an emulsifier, humectant, and fungicide obtained by the action of certain bacteria on glycerol

Direct Reduced Iron (DRI) (V): Reduced Iron.

Disodium inosinate (B): flavor enhancer often derived from meat or fish (sardines). Can also be from vegetable or fungal source.

Down (A): the undercoating of waterfowl (especially ducks and geese). See Feathers.

Duodenum substances (A): from the digestive tracts of cows and pigs. Can be found in vitamin tablets.

Elastin (A): protein uniting muscle fibers in meat

Emu oil (A): oil derived from the rendered fat of the emu, a large Australian flightless bird

Enzymes (B): protein molecules produced by living cells. Act as catalysts in living organisms, regulating the rate of chemical reactions without being changed in the process. Enzymes can be derived from animals, plants, bacteria, fungi, and yeast. Most industrial enzymes consist of a mixture of enzymes. Enzymes include actinidin, amylase, bromelain, catalase, chymotrypsin, ficin, glucose isomerase, lactase, lipase, lipoxygenase, papain, rennet, and trypsin.

Ergocalciferol (B): vitamin D2

Erythorbic Acid (V): food additive used as an antioxidant in processed foods; produced from sucrose.

Estrogen/Estradiol (A): from cow ovaries and pregnant mares' urine

Fatty acids (B): organic compounds: saturated, polyunsaturated and unsaturated

FD&C Colors (B): colors that have been certified safe for use in food, drugs, and cosmetics by the FDA (US Food and Drug Administration). See Colors/Dyes.

FD&C Blue 1 (B): Brilliant Blue FCF. Synthetic dye derived from coal tar. See Colors/Dyes.

FD&C Red 40 (B): Allura Red. Derived from either coal tar or petroleum; not derived from insects. See Colors/Dyes.

FD&C Yellow 5 (B): Tartrazine. Derived from coal tar. See Colors/ Dyes.

FD&C Yellow 6 (B): Monoazo. Derived from coal tar. See Colors/ Dyes.

Feathers (B): epidermal appendage of a bird. Most feathers are removed from birds, especially geese, ducks, or chickens, during slaughter as a by-product of the poultry industry. They can also be plucked from live birds, especially ducks and geese, who are bred for either meat, foie gras, or egg laying and breeding.

Felt (B): cloth made of wool, or of wool and fur or hair

Ferrous Lactate (B): derived from the direct action of lactic acid on iron fillings or from the interaction of calcium lactate with ferrous sulfate

Ferrous Sulfate (V): astringent iron salt obtained in green crystalline form. Used as an antiseptic in cosmetics and in treating anemia in medicine.

Ficin (V): enzyme derived from the latex of the fig tree

Folate (B): vitamin B9

Folic Acid (V): a synthetic form of vitamin B9

Fructose (Syrup) (V): fructose is a sugar found in many fruits, vegetables, and honey. Commercial fructose and fructose-rich syrups are generally produced from starch (almost always corn starch). Sometimes produced from inulin containing plants like chicory roots and Jerusalem artichoke tubers.

Gelatin(e) (A): protein obtained by boiling animal skin, connective tissue or bones, usually from cows or pigs. Edible form of collagen; used as a gelling agent, stabilizer or thickener in cooking. Also used in glues, photographic films, matches, sandpaper, certain soft drinks, playing cards, crepe paper and more.

Glucono delta-lactone (B): also known as gluconolactone or GDL. Fine, white, acidic powder usually produced by the oxidation of glucose by microorganisms.

Gluconolactone (B): glucono delta-lactone

Glucose (B): simple sugar usually produced by hydrolysis of a starch with mineral acids. Starches used include corn, rice, wheat, potato, and arrowroot. Can also be produced synthetically or by adding crystallized cane sugar to a mixture of alcohol and acid. In some countries (like the US), glucose is run through bone-char filters.

Glucose isomerate (V): enzyme derived from the bacteria Streptomyces rubiginosus. Used in the production of fructose syrups (including high fructose corn syrup) by changing glucose into fructose.

Glucosamine (B): dietary supplement used to aid in the relief of joint problems. Usually extracted from the tissues of shellfish. Can also be derived from corn or produced synthetically.

Glycerin(e)/glycerol (B): clear, colorless liquid that is a by-product of the soap-making process obtained by adding alkalies (solutions with a pH greater than 7) to fats and fixed oils. May be derived from animal fats, synthesized from propylene or from fermentation of sugars. Vegetable glycerin is derived from vegetable fats.

Glycine (B): an amino acid, obtainable by hydrolysis of proteins

Guanine/Pearl Essence (A): obtained from scales of fish

Guar Gum (V): gum made from ground guar seeds

Gum Arabic/Gum Acacia (V): natural gum produced by the acacia tree to heal its bark if damaged. Used in cosmetics, candy, syrups, and as glue.

Hide (A): animal skin (raw or tanned)

High Fructose Corn Syrup (HFCS) (V): produced by processing corn starch to yield glucose. This glucose is then treated with enzymes to increase the fructose content to make it sweeter. HFCS contains nearly equal amounts of fructose and glucose. Almost always produced from genetically modified corn.

Honey (A): food made by bees to feed themselves

Hydrochloric Acid (V): formed by heating hydrogen and chlorine gas to form hydrogen chloride gas, which is then absorbed in water

Hydroxypropyl cellulose (V): a derivative of cellulose; used as a thickener in food and for the coating of film and tablets

Hydroxypropyl methylcelluose (HPMC) (V): derived from alkali-treated cellulose that is reacted with methyl chloride and propylene oxide. Can be used as an alternative to gelatin in hard capsules.

Inositol (B): sugar-like dietary supplement of the vitamin B complex. Unofficially referred to as vitamin B8; present in almost all plant and animal tissues. Commercially, it can be obtained from both animal and plant sources (especially corn).

Insulin (B): pancreas of cattle, sheep, or pigs

Inulin (V): a naturally occurring carbohydrate found in the roots and tubers of many plants. Usually extracted from chicory root.

Isinglass (A): very pure form of gelatin obtained from the air bladders of some freshwater fishes, especially the sturgeon

Katsuobushi (okaka) (A): essential ingredient in Japanese cuisine. Made by drying either skipjack tuna or bonito fish into hard blocks and then creating flakes by using a shaving tool. Used as a topping or filling in many Japanese dishes; main ingredient of dashi.

Keratin (A): protein found in hair, hoofs, horns, and feathers

L-cysteine (B): derived from hair, both human and animal, or feathers. Can be synthetically produced from coal tar.

L-cysteine hydrochloride (B): compound produced from L-cysteine

Lactic acid (B): acid produced by the fermentation of whey, cornstarch, potatoes, or molasses

Lactase (V): enzyme derived from fungus of yeast; prevents lactose from being broken down into glucose and galactose. Used in the dairy industry for people who are lactose intolerant.

Lactoflavin (B): vitamin B2.
Lactose (A): milk sugar; type of sugar only found in milk
Lanolin(e) (A): fat extracted from sheep's wool
Lard (A): fat surrounding the stomach and kidneys of pig, sheep, and cattle
Laurel (V): fresh berries and leaf extract of the laurel tree
Lauric Acid (V): constituent of vegetable fats, especially coconut oil and laurel oil. Derivatives are used as a base in the manufacture of soaps, detergents, and lauryl alcohol.
Lauryl Alcohol (V): compound usually produced from coconut oil (which is naturally high in lauric acid) or from a petroleum based version of lauric acid
Leather (A): tanned hide (mostly from cattle but also sheep, pigs and goats, etc.)
Lecithin (B): fatty substance found in nerve tissues, egg yolk, blood, and other tissues. Mainly obtained commercially from soya bean, peanut, and corn.
Limestone (V): porous rock formed over thousands of years from the compression of shells and bones of marine animals
Lipase (B): enzyme from the stomachs, tongue glands of calves, kids, and lambs. Can also be from derived from plants, fungus, or yeast. It breaks down fat to glycerol and fatty acids.
Lipoxygenase (V): enzyme derived from soybeans. It catalyzes the oxidation reaction; used in the baking industry to make bread appear more white.
Lutein (B): substance of deep yellow color found in egg yolk. Obtained commercially from marigold.

Magnesium stearate (B): ester of magnesium and stearic acid
Malic Acid (V): natural acid present in fruits and vegetables. Produced synthetically for use in food products, pharmaceuticals, paints, soaps, and more.
Maltodextrin (V): sugar obtained by hydrolysis of starch
Methanol (V): also known as methyl alcohol or wood alcohol. Used to be produced as a by-product of the destructive distillation of wood. Currently usually produced synthetically.
Methyl alcohol (V): Methanol

Mannitol (Mannite) (V): obtained from the dried sap of the flowering ash or from seaweed

Methyl cellulose (methylcellulose) (V): synthetically produced by heating cellulose with a solution of sodium hydroxide and treating it with methyl chloride. Used as a thickener in sauces and dressings.

Mentha (mint) (V): derived from flowering plants in the mint family

Metafolin (V): brand name for a synthetically produced form of folate, which is chemically identical to the active form of folate found in food. Created by the company, Merck.

Methyl cinnamate (V): derived by heating methanol, cinnamic acid and sulfuric acid

Methyl chloride (chloromethane) (V): colorless, poisonous gas or liquid mostly of natural origin. It is released into the environment from the oceans and is used as a spray for pesticides in food storage and processing.

Milk Sugar (A): Lactose

Mink oil (A): from minks

Modified (food) starch (V): starch treated physically or chemically to modify one or more of its key physical or chemical properties. Physical modification can include drum-drying, extrusion, spray drying, or heat/moisture treatment. Chemicals used to modify starch include propylene oxide, succinic anhydride, 1-octenyl succinic anhydride, aluminum sulfate or sodium hydroxide.

Mohair (A): cloth or yarn made from the hair of the angora goat

Monoazo (Sunset Yellow FCF, Orange Yellow S) (B): FD&C Yellow 6

Monocalcium Phosphate (B): (Monobasic calcium phosphate, Monocalcium orthophosphate); Monobasic form of calcium phosphate

Mono-Diglycerides (B): Emulsifying agents in puddings, ice cream, peanut butter, bread, etc. Can be derived from plants (oils from corn, peanuts or soybeans) or animals (cows and hogs).

Monosodium glutamate (MSG) (V): produced from seaweed or by a bacterial fermentation process with molasses or starch and ammonium salts

Musk (B): substance secreted in a gland or sac by the male musk deer

Natural (B): ingredients are not synthetic or artificial, but extracted directly from either plants or animal products

Natural flavor (B): flavor derived from spices, fruits, fruit juices, vegetables, vegetable juices, plant materials, meat, seafood, poultry, eggs, dairy products or their fermentation products. Significant function of a natural flavor is not nutritional but flavoring.

Natural Red 4 (A): Cochineal

Niacin (B): vitamin B3.

Nicotinic Acid (B): vitamin B3.

NutraSweet (V): aspartame

Nutritional Yeast (B): commercial food product containing deactivated yeast. Sold in the form of yellow powder or flakes. Used as a condiment or food supplement. Often vegan, but some brands use animal products like whey.

Octinoxate (V): also known as octyl methoxycinnamate; Ester of methyl cinnamate

Octyl Methoxycinnamate (V): Octinoxate

Oestrogen (B): female sex hormone from cow ovaries or pregnant mares' urine

Oleic acid (B): fatty acid occurring in animal and vegetable fats

Oleic alcohol (B): oleyl alcohol. Fatty alcohol derived from natural fats and oils, including beef fat and fish oil. Can also be manufactured from esters of oleic acid.

Oleoic oil (A): liquid obtained from pressed tallow

Oleostearin (A): solid obtained from pressed tallow

Oleth-2 through 50 (B): polyethylene glycol ethers of oleic alcohol

Orange Yellow S (B): FD&C Yellow 6

Oxybenzone (V): derived from isopropanol, which is prepared from propylene, obtained in the cracking of petroleum

Palmitate (B): salt or ester of palmitic acid

Palmitic acid (B): fatty acid that occurs in palm oil and most other fats and oils

Panthenol/Dexpanthenol/Vitamin B Complex Factor (B): can come from animal, plant, or synthetic sources

Papain (V): enzyme derived from the unripe fruit of the papaya plant. Used for clearing beverages, added to farina to reduce cooking time; used medically to prevent adhesions.

Paracasein (A): chemical product of the action of rennin or pepsin on casein. To make hard cheese, paracasein is combined with soluble calcium salts to form calcium paracaseinate (cheese curd).

Paraffin (V): waxy substance obtained from distillates of wood, coal, petroleum, or shale oil

Parchment (B): skin of the sheep or goat, dressed and prepared for writing, etc.

Pearl (A): concretion of layers of pain-dulling nacre formed around a foreign particle within the shell of various bivalve molluscs, principally the oyster

Pectin (V): a substance found in the primary cell walls and the non-woody parts of plants. Used as a gelling agent, thickener, and stabilizer in food. Commercially, obtained mostly from dried citrus peels and apples as a by-product of juice production.

PEG (B): abbreviation of polyethylene glycol or polyoxyethylene glycol; polymeric forms of ethylene oxide. Can be either synthetic or derived from animal or vegetable sources.

Pepsin (A): enzyme usually derived from the stomach of grown calves or sometimes pigs.

Petroleum (V): oily, flammable liquid composed of a complex mixture of hydrocarbons occurring in many places in the upper strata of the earth. A fossil fuel believed to have originated from both plant and animal sources millions of years ago.

Pharmaceutical Glaze (A): Resinous Glaze.

Phenol (V): obtained from coal tar

Phosphoric Acid (V): inorganic acid produced by reacting ground phosphate rock with sulfuric acid

Placenta (A): organ by which the fetus is attached to the umbilical cord
Polyethylene (V): a product of petroleum gas or dehydration of alcohol
Polyglycerol polyricinoleate (B): produced from castor oil and glycerol esters
Polysorbate 60 (B): a condensate of sorbitol with stearic acid
Polysorbate 80 (B): a condensate of sorbitol and oleic acid
Polyvinylpyrrolidone (PVP) (V): a water-soluble polymer from synthetic origin. Used in products like pharmaceutical tablets, shampoo, toothpaste, batteries, paint, and adhesives.
Polyoxyethylene (8) stearate (B): a mixture of stearate and ethylene oxide
Polyoxyethylene (40) stearate (B): a mixture of stearate and ethylene oxide produced by a reaction of ethylene oxide with stearic acid
Potassium Chloride (V): occurs naturally as the mineral sylvite and found combined in many minerals and in brines and ocean water
Potassium Hydroxide (V): obtained commercially from the electrolysis of potassium chloride solution
Potassium Lactate (B): potassium salt of lactic acid
Potassium Sorbate (V): ascorbic acid potassium salt. Manufactured by neutralization of ascorbic acid with potassium hydroxide.
Progesterone (B): sex hormone
Propolis (A): bee glue; used by bees to stop up crevices and fix combs to the hive
Propylene/propene (V): flammable gas obtained by cracking petroleum
Propylene glycol (B): 1,2-propylene glycol; propane-1,2-diol. Manufactured by treating propylene with chlorinated water, then treating with sodium carbonate solution or by heating glycerol with sodium hydroxide and distilling the mixture.
Propylene/propene oxide (V): flammable liquid, derived from propylene

Quinoline Yellow (B): obtained by the interaction of aniline with acetaldehyde and formaldehyde or by distillation of coal tar, bones, and alkaloids

Reduced Iron (V): also known as Direct Reduced Iron (DRI) or Sponge Iron. Used to fortify foods, like flour. Produced from either iron ore or mill scale (the surface of hot rolled steel) by reduction with hydrogen or carbon monoxide.

Rennet (B): extract usually obtained from a newly-born calf stomach. Rennet contains the enzymes rennin and a little amount of pepsin. The older the veal calf, the more pepsin will be found in the rennet. Rennet can also be derived from synthetic sources or from bacteria and fungus

Rennin (B): enzyme found in rennet. Used to split the casein molecule during cheese making to clot milk and turn it into curds and whey.

Red 40 (B): FD&C Red 40

Resinous Glaze (A): also known as pharmaceutical glaze, confectioner's glaze, pure food glaze, and natural glaze. Made from various types of food grade shellac. Also known as beetle juice, even though the lac insect it's derived from is a scale insect and not a beetle.

Reticulin (A): one of the structural elements (together with elastin and collagen) of skeletal muscle

Riboflavin (B): vitamin B2

Riboflavin-5-Phosphate (B): more soluble form of riboflavin

Roe (A): eggs obtained from the abdomen of slaughtered female fish

Royal jelly (A): food on which bee larvae are fed which causes them to develop into queen bees

Sable (A): fur from the sable marten, a small carnivorous mammal

Salicylic Acid (V): derived from the leaves of wintergreen, meadowsweet, willow bark, or other plants. Can also be produced synthetically by heating phenol with carbon dioxide.

Shellac (A): insect secretion

Silk (A): cloth made from the fiber produced by the larvae ("silk worm") of certain bombycine moths, the harvesting of which entails the destruction of the insect

Sodium Alginate (V): sodium salt of alginic acid extracted from brown seaweed

Sodium Aluminum Sulfate (V): white solid used as an acidity regulator in foods. Mainly used in the manufacturing of baking powder. Produced by combining sodium sulfate and aluminum sulfate.

Sodium Benzoate (V): sodium salt of benzoic acid. Produced by reacting sodium hydroxide with benzoic acid. Used as a food preservative.

Sodium Bicarbonate/Baking Soda (V): bicarbonate of Soda

Sodium Carbonate (V): Soda Ash; a sodium salt of carbonic acid

Sodium Chloride (V): chemical term for table salt. Can be mined (rock salt), obtained by adding water to salt deposits (evaporated salt), or obtained from oceans and salt lakes (sea salt).

Sodium Hydroxide (V): Caustic Soda. A water-soluble solid usually produced by processing salt water. Used to be obtained from the ashes of a certain kind of seaweed.

Sodium Lactate (B): sodium salt of lactic acid

Sodium Laureth Sulfate (SLES) (V): sodium salt of sulfated ethoxylated lauryl alcohol

Sodium Lauryl Sulfate (SLS) (V): prepared by sulfation of lauryl alcohol followed by neutralization with sodium carbonate

Sodium Metabisulfite (V): inorganic salt. White to yellowish powder with sulfur dioxide odor. Used as a disinfectant, antioxidant, and preservative.

Sodium Phosphate (mono-, di-, and tri-) (V): synthetic material generally prepared by the partial or total neutralization of phosphoric acid using sodium carbonate or sodium hydroxide

Sodium stearoyl-2-lactylate (B): prepared from lactic acid and fatty acids

Sodium Sulfate (V): sodium salt of sulfuric acid

Sorbic acid (V): white powder obtained from fruit or produced synthetically

Sorbitan monolaurate (V): derived from raw materials of vegetable origin. Commercially known as Span 20.

Sorbitan monostearate (B): manufactured by reacting stearic acid with sorbitol to yield a mixture of esters. Commercially known as Span 60

Sorbitan monooleate (B): derived from animal or vegetable sources. Commercially known as Span 80. Vegetable-derived version known as Span 80V.

Sorbitan monopalmitate (V): derived from raw materials of vegetable origin. Commercially known as Span 40.

Sorbitan tristearate (B): derived from animal or vegetable sources. Commercially known as Span 65. Vegetable-derived version known as Span 65V.

Sorbitan Trioleate (B): derived from animal or vegetable sources. Commercially known as Span 85. Vegetable-derived version known as Span 85V.

Sorbitol (V): sugar alcohol derived from fruit like cherries, plums, pears, apples, or from corn, seaweed, and algae

Sourdough starter (B): also known as "starter culture," "sourdough culture," or "sour culture." Usually made with a mixture of flour and water inhabited by yeast and lacto bacteria containing no animal ingredients. Sometimes yogurt is used in the starter. Bread made from a sourdough culture is called sourdough bread.

Sperm oil (A): oil found in the head of the various species of whales

Spermaceti (A): fatty substance derived as a wax from the head of the sperm whale

Sponge (B): aquatic animal or colony of animals of a "low order," characterized by a tough elastic skeleton of interlaced fibers

Sponge Iron (V): Reduced Iron

Squalene/squalane (B): found in the liver of the shark (and rats)

Starch (V): complex carbohydrate found in seeds, fruits, tubers, roots and stem pith of plants such as corn, potatoes, wheat, beans, and rice

Stearate (B): salt of stearic acid

Stearic acid (B): fat from cows, pigs, sheep, dogs, or cats. Can be obtained from vegetable sources.

Stearin(e) (B): general name for the three glycerids (monostearin, distearin, tristearin). Formed by the combination of stearic acid and glycerin, chiefly applied to tristearin, the main constituent of tallow or suet

Stearyl alcohol (B): prepared from sperm whale oil or vegetable sources

Stearyl tartrate (Stearyl palmityl tartrate)(B): made from stearyl alcohol and tartaric acid

Sucroglycerides (B): obtained by reacting sucrose with an edible fat or oil with or without the presence of a solvent

Sucralose (B): known under the brand name Splenda. Produced from cane sugar. Some but not all Splenda producers have confirmed they don't use bone char as a filter. Sucralose is tested on animals.

Sucrose (B): Sugar

Suede (B): kid, pig, or calf skin tanned

Suet (B): solid fat prepared from the kidneys of cattle and sheep

Sugar (B): a sweet crystallizable material that consists wholly or essentially of sucrose. Obtained commercially from sugarcane or sugar beet. Beet sugar is vegan, but some cane sugars are processed through boneblack.

Sulfur Dioxide (V): toxic, colorless gas formed primarily by the combustion of sulfur-containing material, like fossil fuels

Sulfuric Acid (V): oil of vitriol; highly corrosive acid usually produced from sulfur dioxide

Sunette (V): Acesulfame

Sunset Yellow FCF (B): FD&C Yellow 6

Synthetic (V): produced by chemical synthesis, which means that parts or elements are combined to form a whole. Unlike artificial products, synthetic products are made from ingredients that do not occur (independently) in nature.

Tallow (A): hard animal fat, especially that obtained from the parts about the kidneys of ruminating animals

Tartaric Acid (V): an organic acid present in many fruits, especially in grapes. Usually obtained as a by-product of wine making.

Tartrazine (B): FD&C Yellow 5

TBHQ (Tertiary Butylhydroquinone) (V): synthetic food preservative used in oils, margarines, crackers, fast foods, and many other food products. Produced from phenol and butane.

Tertiary Butyl hydroquinone (V): TBHQ

Testosterone (B): male hormone

Thiamine Mononitrate (V): synthetic form of vitamin B1; synthesized by removing a chloride ion from thiamine hydrochloride and mixing it with nitric acid.

Thiamine Hydrocholide (V): synthetic form of vitamin B1. Produced from coal tar, ammonia, acetone and hydrochloric acid.

Toluene (V): a colorless liquid hydrocarbon derived from petroleum processing

Tricalcium Phosphate (B): (Calcium phosphate, tribasic) tribasic form of calcium phosphate. Also known as calcium orthophosphate. Consists of a mixture of calcium phosphates.

Tocopherols (V): vitamin E

Trypsin (A): enzyme usually derived from porcine pancreas

Turmeric (V): East Indian perennial herb

Urea (B): also known as carbamide; waste product of digested protein filtered out by the kidneys and excreted from the body in urine. Commercially, almost always produced from synthetic ammonia and carbon dioxide. Rarely produced from animal urine.

Vegetable Carbon (B): derived from either burnt vegetable matter, incomplete combustion of natural gas, activated charcoal, bones, blood, meat, or various fats oils and resins

Vegetable Glycerin (V): Glycerin derived from vegetable fats

Vellum (B): fine parchment prepared from the skins of calves, lambs, or kids

Velvet (B): fabric made usually of silk but also rayon or nylon

Vitamin A (retinol) (B): aliphatic alcohol. Some possible sources are fish liver oil, egg yolks, butter, lemongrass, carrots, or synthetics.

Vitamin B1 (Thiamine, Thiamin) (B): used to fortify foods or as a supplement. Two of the synthetic forms are known as thiamine mononitrate and thiamine hydrochloride.

Vitamin B2 (Riboflavin, Lactoflavin) (B): used as a food coloring, to fortify foods, or as a supplement. Produced synthetically or by a fermentation process with genetically modified Bacillus subtilis. Usually vegan, but in rare cases it can be produced from animal sources like beef, especially when marked as being "natural."

Vitamin B3 (Niacin, Nicotinic Acid) (B): used as a cholesterol treatment, to fortify foods, or as a supplement. The largest commercial use is to fortify animal feed. Usually produced synthetically. In rare cases it can be derived from animal sources.

Vitamin B9 (Folic Acid, Folate) (B): used to fortify foods or as a supplement, especially for pregnant women. Usually produced synthetically. Folate is the general term for Vitamin B9, whereas folic acid refers to the synthetic compound used in supplements and food fortification.

Vitamin C (V): Ascorbic acid

Vitamin D2 (Ergocalciferol) (B): vitamin usually derived from plant sterols or yeast. Can also be derived from animal fats.

Vitamin D3 (Cholecalciferol) (B): vitamin usually derived from animal sources like lanolin, milk, egg yolk, and fish liver oil. Can also be derived from microbial or synthetic sources. Please note that synthetic vitamin D3 can have an animal ingredient as their starting raw material.

Vitamin E (V): natural-source vitamin E (d-alpha-tocopherol) is obtained by distillation of vegetable oils (primarily from soya beans, rapeseed and sunflower); synthetic, chemically manufactured vitamin E (dl-alpha-tocopherol) is a mixture of eight diastereoisomers in equal proportions.

Volaise (A): ostrich meat

Waxy maze (V): corn starch; sticky material from the inside of the corn kernel

Waxed Paper (B): often coated with paraffin or tallow. Waxed paper from the companies If You Care (100% soybean wax) and Natural Value (100% paraffin) are vegan.

Whey (A): residue from milk after the removal of the casein and most of the fat; by-product of cheese making

White Mineral Oil (V): obtained from petroleum and used in baked goods

Wool (A): hair forming the fleecy coat of the domesticated sheep (and similar animals)

Xanthan gum (corn sugar gum) (V): gum produced by the fermentation of corn sugar with the microbe Xanthomonas campestris

Yeast (V): microscopic unicellular fungus; different yeast products include baker's yeast, nutritional yeast, and brewer's yeast.

Yellow 5 (B): FD&C Yellow 5

Yellow 6 (B): FD&C Yellow 6

E Numbers

E100 (V): Curcumin

E101 (B): Riboflavin, vitamin B2

E101a (B): Riboflavin-5-Phosphate

E102 (B): Tartrazine, FD&C Yellow 5

E104 (B): Quinoline Yellow

E110 (B): Sunset Yellow FCF, Orange Yellow S, FD&C Yellow 6, Monoao

E120 (A): Carminic acid, Carmine, Natural Red 4, Cochineal

E129 (B): Allura Red, FD&C Red 40

E133 (B): Brilliant Blue FCF, FD&C Blue 1

E150a (B): plain caramel; manufactured by heating carbohydrates with or without acids or alkalis

E150b (B): caustic caramel; produced like E150a, but in the presence of sulfite compounds

E150c (B): ammonia caramel; produced like E150a, but in the presence of ammonium compounds

E150d (B): sulfite ammonia caramel; produced like E150a, but with both sulfite and ammonium compounds

E153 (B): Carbon Black, Vegetable Carbon

E160a (V): Carotene. Note: gelatin may be used as a stabilizer. See beta carotene.

E160b (V): Annatto, bixin, norbixin

E160c (V): Capsanthin, capsorubin, Paprika extract. Extracted from the fruit pod and seeds of the red pepper.

E162 (V): Beetroot Red, Betanin; natural extract from beetroot

E163 (V): Anthocyanins

E170 (B): Calcium Carbonate, Chalk
E200 (V): Sorbic Acid
E202 (V): Potassium Sorbate
E211 (V): Sodium Benzoate
E223 (V): Sodium Metabisulfite
E270 (B): Lactic acid
E296 (V): Malic Acid
E300 (V): Ascorbic Acid, vitamin C
E315 (V): Erythorbic Acid
E322 (B): Lecithin
E325 (B): Sodium Lactate
E326 (B): Potassium Lactate
E327 (B): Calcium Lactate
E341 (B): Calcium Phosphate
E375 (B): Vitamin B3
E385 (V): Calcium Disodium EDTA
E406 (V): Agar, agar-agar
E407 (V): Carrageenan
E412 (V): Guar gum
E415 (V): Xanthan gum
E420 (V): Sorbitol
E421 (V): Mannitol
E422 (B): Glycerin(e), Glycerol
E430 (B): Polyoxyethylene (8) stearate
E431 (B): Polyoxyethylene (40) stearate
E432 (B): Polyoxyethylene (20) sorbitan monolaurate, Polysorbate 20
E433 (B): Polyoxyethylene (20) sorbitan monooleate, Polysorbate 80
E434 (B): Polyoxyethylene (20) sorbitan monopalmitate, Polysorbate 40
E435 (B): Polyoxyethylene (20) sorbitan monostearate, Polysorbate 60
E436 (B): Polyoxyethylene (20) sorbitan tristearate, Polysorbate 65
E441 (A): Gelatin
E470(a)(B): Sodium, potassium and calcium salts of fatty acids
E470(b) (B): Magnesium salts of fatty acids
E471 (B): Mono- and diglycerides of fatty acids, Glyceryl monostearate, Glyceryl distearate
E472(a) (B): Acetic acid esters of mono- and diglycerides of fatty acids

E472(b) (B): Lactic acid esters of mono- and diglycerides of fatty acids
E472(c) (B): Citric acid esters of mono- and diglycerides of fatty acids
E472(d) (B): Tartaric acid esters of mono- and diglycerides of fatty acids
E472(e) (B): Mono- and diacetyl tartaric acid esters of mono- and diglycerides of fatty acids
E472(f) (B): Mixed acetic and tartaric acid esters of mono- and diglycerides of fatty acids
E473 (B): Sucrose esters of fatty acids
E474 (B): Sucroglycerides
E475 (B): Polyglycerol esters of fatty acids
E476 (B): Polyglycerol polyricinoleate
E477 (B): Propane-1, 2-diol esters of fatty acids, propylene glycol esters of fatty acids
478 (B): Lactylated fatty acid esters of glycerol and propane-1
E479(b) (B): Thermally oxidized soya bean oil interacted with mono- and diglycerides of fatty acids
E481 (B): Sodium stearoyl-2-lactylate
E482 (B): Calcium stearoyl-2-lactylate
E483 (B): Stearyl tartrate
E491 (B): Sorbitan monostearate
E492 (B): Sorbitan tristearate
E493 (V): Sorbitan monolaurate
E494 (B): Sorbitan monooleate
E495 (V): Sorbitan monopalmitate
E507 (V): Hydrochloric Acid
E508 (V): Potassium Chloride
E521(V): Sodium Aluminum Sulfate
E526 (V): Calcium Hydroxide.
E542 (A): Bone phosphate
E570 (B): Stearic acid
E572 (B): Magnesium stearate, calcium stearate
E585 (B): Ferrous lactate
E621 (V): Monosodium glutamate (MSG)
E631 (A): Disodium inosinate

E640 (B): Glycine and its sodium salt
E901 (B): Beeswax
E902 (V): Candelilla wax
E903 (V): Carnauba wax
E904 (A): Shellac
E910 (B): L-cysteine
E913 (A): Lanolin
E920 (B): L-cysteine hydrochloride
E950 (V): Acesulfame
E1201 (V): Polyvinylpyrrolidone
E1400 (V): Dextrin

This extensive list was contributed by Wanda Embar, Vegan Peace; www.veganpeace.com.

Notes

Chapter 1

1. Andrea Hayley, "How the American Diet Sets a Bad Example for the World," *Epoch Times,* May 7, 2016.

Chapter 2

1. Cheryl Long and Tabitha Alterman, "Meet Real Free-Range Eggs," *Mother Earth News,* October/November 2007. http://www.motherearthnews.com/real-food/free-range-eggs-zmaz07onzgoe, accessed January 19, 2017.
2. "The Protein Myth," Physicians Committee for Responsible Medicine;http://www.pcrm.org/health/diets/vsk/vegetarian-starter-kit-protein; accessed January 19, 2017.
3. World Health Organization, Press Release No. 240, October 26, 2015.
4. Dr. Russell Blaylock, MD, "High-Protein Diet Dangers," *News Max Health,* December 13, 2010.
5. Agatha M. Thrash, MD, "Dangers of a High Protein Diet," September 15, 2013; http://www.ucheepines.org/dangers-of-a-high-protein-diet/; accessed January 19, 2017.

Chapter 5

1. Stephen Parcell, "Sulfur in human nutrition and applications in medicine," US National Library of Medicine, National Institutes of Health, Altern Med Rev (February 7, 2002); https://www.ncbi.nlm.nih.gov/pubmed/11896744; accessed January 23, 2017.

2. M. Anke, B. Groppel, H. Kronemann, M. Grün, "Nickel—an essential element," National Library of Medicine, National Institutes of Health 1984; (53):339-65.

3. Ibid.

Chapter 7

1. Health Matters Program (2011); "Water Amounts in Fruits and Vegetables," adapted from Water Content of Fruits and Vegetables prepared by Sandra Bastin, Foods and Nutrition Specialist, and Kim Henken, Extension Associate for ENRI. Information taken from Bowes & Church's Food Values, 1994.

2. *United States Environmental Protection Agency;*https://www.epa.gov/sites/production/files/2015-11documents/2005_09_14_faq_fs_homewatertesting.pdf;accessedJanuary 19, 2017.

Chapter 8

1. Friedrich Manz, MD and Thomas Remer, PhD, "PRAL List," *Journal of the American Dietetic Association,* July 1995, Volume 95, Number 7, pp 791-797.

2. Alesia Lucas, "Meet Azodicarbonamide," SaferChemicals.org, October 20, 2014; http://saferchemicals.org/2014/10/20/meet-azodicarbonamide/; accessed January 23, 2017.

Chapter 10

1. Seth J. Wechsler, "Recent Trends in GE Adoption," United States Department of Agriculture Economic Research Service, November 3, 2016.

2. "Products that use Corn"; https://healthhabits.files.wordpress.com/2009/01/products-that-use-corn.pdf; accessed January 20, 2017.

Chapter 12

1. http://www.medicinenet.com/script/main/art.asp?article key=31372; accessed January 21, 2017.

Chapter 13

1. Mohamad Sleiman, Jennifer M. Logue, V. Nahuel Montesinos, Marion L. Russell, Marta I. Litter, Lara A. Gundel, and Hugo Destaillats, "Emissions from Electronic Cigarettes: Key Parameters Affecting the Release of Harmful Chemicals," *Environmental Science & Technology,* July 27, 2016; http://pubs.acs.org/doi/abs/10.1021/acs.est.6b01741; accessed January 21, 2017.
2. Dr. Otto Warburg lecture, June 30, 1966; http://thewebmatrix.net/organicsulfurstudy/CauseofCancer-LecturebyDr.Otto Warburg-deliveredtoNobelLaureates.pdf;accessedJanuary 21,2017. Note: Bold emphasis is the author's, not the lecturer's.
3. Cancer Fact sheet No. 297, updated February 2015, World Health Organization;http://www.who.int/mediacentre/factsheets/fs297/en/; accessed January 21, 2017.

Chapter 16

1. Melinda Smith, MA, Lawrence Robinson, and Jeanne Segal, PhD; reviewed by Anna Glezer, MD, "Anxiety Medication What You Need to Know About Anti-Anxiety Drugs";HelpGuide.Org, updated December 2016; http://www.helpguide.org/articles/anxiety/anxiety-medication.htm; accessed January 21,2017. http://www.helpguide.org/articles/ anxiety/anxiety-medication.htm
2. "Lyrica Side Effects," Drugs.com; https://www.drugs.com/sfx/lyrica-side-effects.html; accessed January 21, 2017.

Chapter 17

1. "Cardiovascular diseases (CVDs)," World Health Organization; http://www.who.int/mediacentre/factsheets/fs317/en/; accessed January 21, 2017.
2. "Heart Disease Facts," Centers for Disease Control and Prevention; http://www.cdc.gov/HeartDisease/facts.htm; accessed January 21, 2017.
3. Ibid.

Chapter 19

1. The National Institute of Diabetes and Digestive and Kidney Diseases of The National Institutes of Health, "Your Kidneys and How They Work," *NIH Publication: 98-4241,* March 1998; http://www.niddk.nih.gov/health/kidney/pubs/yourkids/index.htm; accessed January 21, 2017.

Chapter 20

1. Leslie Mann, "Study finds nearly half of Americans not drinking enough water," Special to the *Chicago Tribune,* June 5, 2013; http://articles.chicagotribune.com/2013-06-05/health/ct-x-0605-drinking-water-20130605_1_dietary-guidelines-much-water-drinking-water;accessed January 21, 2017.

Chapter 21

1. International Agency for Research on Cancer, World Health Organization Press Release No. 240, October 26, 2015; www.iarc.fr/en/media-centre/pr/2015/pdfs/pr240_E.pdf; accessed January 31, 2017.
2. Dr. Joseph Mercola, "Soy: This 'Miracle Health Food' Has Been Linked to Brain Damage and Breast Cancer," September 18, 2010;http://articles.mercola.com/sites/articles/archive/2010/09/18/soy-can-damage-your-health.aspx;accessedJanuary 22, 2017.

Chapter 22

1. B. N. Singh and Shankar S. Krivastava, "Green tea catechin, epigallocatechin-3-gallate (EGCG): mechanisms, perspectives and clinical applications," US Library of Medicine, National Institutes for Health, 2011; http://www.ncbi.nlm.nih.gov/pubmed/21827739; accessed January 21, 2017.

Chapter 24

1. Jessica Firger, "CDC warns of common parasites plaguing million in U.S.," CBSNEWS, May 8, 2014; http://www.cbsnews.com/news/parasites-causing-infections-in-the-us-cdc-says/; accessed January 21, 2017. http://www.cbsnews.com/news/parasites-causing-infections-in-the-us-cdc-says/
2. "Parasites—Neglected Parasitic Infections," Center for Disease Control and Prevention, https://www.cdc.gov/parasites/npi/index.html; accessed January 21, 2017.
3. "Health and Safety Precautions in the Dominican Republic," DominicanRepublic24.com; http://www.dominicanrepublic24.com/healthandsafety.html; accessed January 22, 2017. http://www.dominicanrepublic24.com/healthandsafety.html

   https://www.epa.gov/sites/production/files/201511/documents/2005_09_14_faq_fs_homewatertesting.pdf

Bibliography

Alterman, Tabitha and Cheryl Long. "Meet Real Free-Range Eggs," *Mother Earth News* (October/November 2007).

Anke, M., B. Groppel, H. Kronemann, and M. Grün. "Nickel—an essential element," National Library of Medicine, National Institutes of Health (1984): (53):339-65.

Blaylock, Russell, MD. "High-Protein Diet Dangers," *NewsMax Health* (December 13, 2010).

Cancer Fact sheet No. 297, World Health Organization (February 2015).

Decuypere, Jeanne, DC. "Nutrition Charts," Health-Alternatives.com (2016).

Destaillats, Hugo, et al. "Emissions from Electronic Cigarettes: Key Parameters Affecting the Release of Harmful Chemicals," American Chemical Society Environmental Science and Technology (July 27, 2016).

"Diabetes: Carbohydrate Food List," University of Michigan Diabetes Education Program (April 2012).

Embar, Wanda. "Ingredients," VeganPeace.com (2016).

"Examples of population-wide interventions that can be implemented to reduce CVDs," World Health Organization (2015).

Firger, Jessica. "CDC warns of common parasites plaguing millions in U.S.," *CBS News* (May 8, 2014)

Friedrich Manz, MD, and Thomas Remer, PhD. "PRAL List," *Journal of the American Dietetic Association* (July 1995, Volume 95, Number 7, 791-797).

Hayley, Andrea. "How the American Diet Sets a Bad Example for the World," *Epoch Times* (May 7, 2016).

"Health & Safety Precautions in the Dominican Republic," DominicanRepublic24.com (2016).

"Heart Disease Facts," Center for Disease Control and Prevention (August 10, 2015).

"Home Water Testing," United States Environmental Protection Agency (May 2005).

Henken, Kim and Sandra Bastin. "Water Content of Fruits and Vegetables," Bowes & Church's Food Values (1994).

Lucas, Alesia. "Meet Aodicarbonamide," SaferChemicals.org (October 20, 2014).

"Lyrica side effects," Drugs.com (August 2012).

Mann, Leslie. "Study finds nearly half of Americans not drinking enough water," *Chicago Tribune* (June 5, 2013).

MedTerms (CPAP), MedicineNet.com (October 30, 2013).

Mercola, MD, Joseph. "Soy: This 'Miracle Health Food' Has Been Linked to Brain Damage and Breast Cancer" (September 18, 2010).

"Parasites–Neglected Parasitic Infections," Center for Disease Control and Prevention, Global Health, Division of Parasitic Disease and Malaria (December 5, 2016).

Parcell, S. "Sulfur in human nutrition and applications in medicine," US Library of Medicine, National Institute for Health (February 7, 2002).

Physicians Committee for Responsible Medicine, "The Protein Myth: Products that use corn," Health Habits (January 2009).

Smith, Melinda, MA, Lawrence Robinson, and Jeanne Segal, PhD. "Anxiety Medication: What You Need to Know About Anti-Anxiety Drugs," HelpGuide.Org (December 2016).

Thrash, MD, Agatha M. "Dangers of a High Protein Diet," Uchee Pines (September 15, 2013).

United States Department of Agriculture, Agricultural Research Service, Nutrient Data Laboratory. "USDA National Nutrient Database for Standard Reference, Release 18" (Version Current: August 2016).

United States Department of Agriculture, Agricultural Research Service, Nutrient Data Laboratory. "United States Department of Agriculture National Nutrient Database for Standard Reference, Release 28." (Version Current: September 2015, slightly revised May 2016).

Wechsler, Seth J. "Recent Trends in GE Adoption," United States Department of Agriculture Economic Research Service (November 3, 2016).

"Your Kidneys and How They Work," NIH Publication: 98-4241, The National Institute of Diabetes and Digestive and Kidney Diseases of The National Institutes of Health (March 1998).